STATISTICS IN PRACTICE

Human and Biological Sciences

Brown and Prescott · Applied Mixed Models in Medicine
Ellenberg, Fleming and DeMets · Data Monitoring Committees in Clinical Trials: A Practical Perspective
Lawson, Browne and Vidal Rodeiro · Disease Mapping With WinBUGS and MLwiN
Lui · Statistical Estimation of Epidemiological Risk
*Marubini and Valsecchi · Analysing Survival Data from Clinical Trials and Observation Studies
Parmigiani · Modeling in Medical Decision Making: A Bayesian Approach
Senn · Cross-over Trials in Clinical Research, *Second Edition*
Senn · Statistical Issues in Drug Development
Spiegelhalter, Abrams and Myles · Bayesian Approaches to Clinical Trials and Health-Care Evaluation
Turner · New Drug Development: Design, Methodology, and Analysis
Whitehead · Design and Analysis of Sequential Clinical Trials, *Revised Second Edition*
Whitehead · Meta-Analysis of Controlled Clinical Trials

Earth and Environmental Sciences

Buck, Cavanagh and Litton · Bayesian Approach to Interpreting Archaeological Data
Glasbey and Horgan · Image Analysis in the Biological Sciences
Helsel · Nondetects and Data Analysis: Statistics for Censored Environmental Data
McBride · Using Statistical Methods for Water Quality Management: Issues, Problems and Solutions
Webster and Oliver · Geostatistics for Environmental Scientists

Industry, Commerce and Finance

Aitken and Taroni · Statistics and the Evaluation of Evidence for Forensic Scientists, *Second Edition*
Brandimarte · Numerical Methods in Finance and Economics: A MATLAB-Based Introduction, *Second Edition*
Brandimarte and Zotteri · Introduction to Distribution Logistics
Chan and Wong · Simulation Techniques in Financial Risk Management
Lehtonen and Pahkinen · Practical Methods for Design and Analysis of Complex Surveys, *Second Edition*
Ohser and Mücklich · Statistical Analysis of Microstructures in Materials Science

*Now available in paperback.

New Drug Development

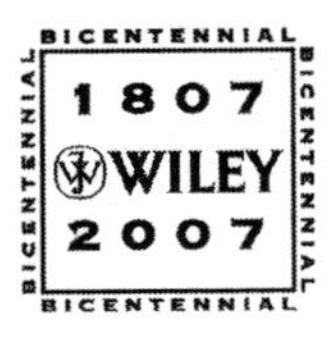

THE WILEY BICENTENNIAL–KNOWLEDGE FOR GENERATIONS

Each generation has its unique needs and aspirations. When Charles Wiley first opened his small printing shop in lower Manhattan in 1807, it was a generation of boundless potential searching for an identity. And we were there, helping to define a new American literary tradition. Over half a century later, in the midst of the Second Industrial Revolution, it was a generation focused on building the future. Once again, we were there, supplying the critical scientific, technical, and engineering knowledge that helped frame the world. Throughout the 20th Century, and into the new millennium, nations began to reach out beyond their own borders and a new international community was born. Wiley was there, expanding its operations around the world to enable a global exchange of ideas, opinions, and know-how.

For 200 years, Wiley has been an integral part of each generation's journey, enabling the flow of information and understanding necessary to meet their needs and fulfill their aspirations. Today, bold new technologies are changing the way we live and learn. Wiley will be there, providing you the must-have knowledge you need to imagine new worlds, new possibilities, and new opportunities.

Generations come and go, but you can always count on Wiley to provide you the knowledge you need, when and where you need it!

WILLIAM J. PESCE
PRESIDENT AND CHIEF EXECUTIVE OFFICER

PETER BOOTH WILEY
CHAIRMAN OF THE BOARD

New Drug Development

Design, Methodology, and Analysis

J. Rick Turner
Department of Clinical Research
Campbell University School of Pharmacy
Morrisville, North Carolina

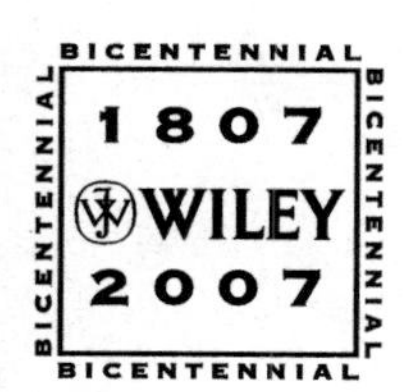

WILEY-INTERSCIENCE
A John Wiley & Sons, Inc., Publication

Published by John Wiley & Sons, Inc., Hoboken, New Jersey.
Published simultaneously in Canada.

Wiley Bicentennial Logo: Richard J. Pacifico

Library of Congress Cataloging-in-Publication Data:

Turner, J. Rick.
New drug development : design, methodology, and analysis / J. Rick Turner.
p.; cm.
Includes bibliographical references and index.
ISBN 978-0-470-07373-5 (cloth : alk. paper)
1. Drug development. 2. Pharmacy. I. Title.
[DNLM: 1. Clinical Trials. 2. Pharmaceutical Preparations—chemical Synthesis. 3. Drug Industry—methods. 4. Statistics. QV 771 T948n 2007]
RS189.T8779 2007
615'.19—dc22 2007008032

Printed in the United States of America.

10 9 8 7 6 5 4 3 2 1

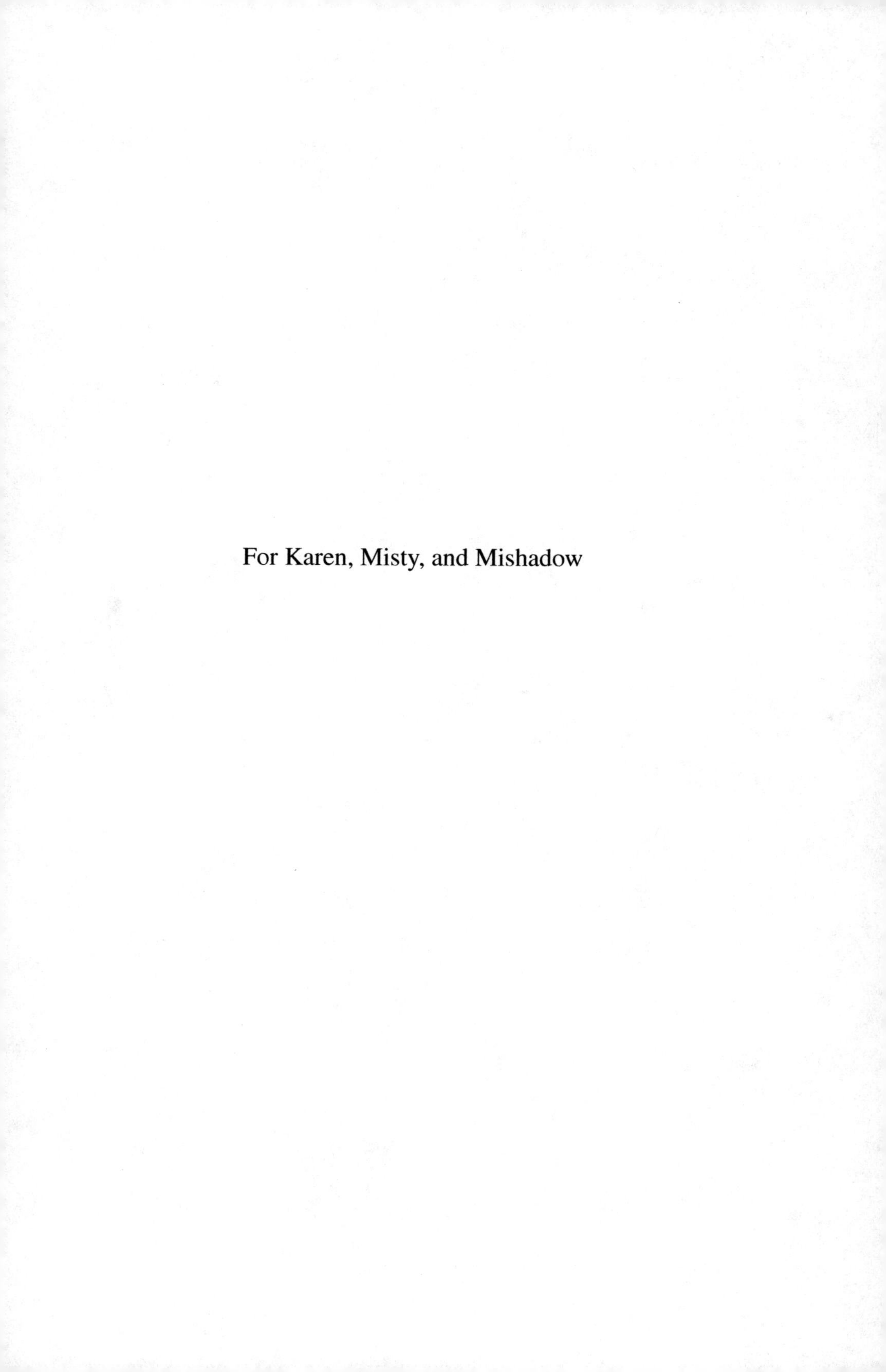

For Karen, Misty, and Mishadow

Contents

Foreword

While passion in any worthwhile pursuit is to be commended, passion about a process that affects the lives of many millions of people throughout the world is particularly so. Pharmaceutical products improve health and quality of life on a scale that is unrivaled by any other medical intervention. Before these drugs are prescribed by physicians, they go through an extremely rigorous process that investigates their safety and their efficacy: This is the process of new drug development.

This investigation is conducted under the governance of regulatory agencies throughout the world. In the United States, the Food and Drug Administration (FDA) shoulders this responsibility. Nonclinical investigation in animals and clinical investigation in humans must be conducted in a specified manner, and all results must be submitted to the FDA in appropriately formatted documentation to achieve marketing approval. At the heart of this investigation and documentation is research methodology, addressed in this volume via discussion of its constituent components of study design, experimental methodology, and statistical analysis.

Dr Turner's exposition is deceptively simple: Successful new drug development requires the integration of careful study design, careful experimental methodology, and careful statistical analysis and interpretation. That is, a clinical trial requires a design that is capable of answering a carefully constructed research question, collection of optimum quality data, the use of appropriate statistical analysis, and interpretation of the numerical results in the context of the research question. Who would doubt the veracity of this position? Unfortunately, while researchers in this field are very likely to agree in spirit, research in new drug development too often does not conform to these simple ideals. Yet, attempting to conduct a research study without full and prior consideration of study design, experimental methodology, and statistical analysis would not be unlike attempting to pilot an airliner without due consideration of the type of aircraft flown (design), its intended destination and route of flight (methodology), and how information gathered in flight will be assessed and incorporated to achieve a safe and successful outcome (analysis) before filling the plane with passengers (study subjects) and departing. Such a flight would almost certainly have a highly unfavorable outcome, with little likelihood of successfully arriving at its intended destination. So too would a research study that was hastily designed and executed without full consideration and implementation of the fundamentals of clinical research so eloquently presented in this book.

From the scientific perspective, an inappropriate study design is generally incapable of answering a research question, no matter how careful the subsequent methodology and analysis. Additionally, the perfect design will not provide optimum information if the research methodology is flawed or an inappropriate statistical analysis is conducted. From the ethical perspective, research subjects voluntarily take part in clinical trials with the understanding that their participation will provide information that is useful and generalizable to a much larger group of people. This is one of the "benefits" that is weighed against the "risks" of their being exposed to a drug under development. If the clinical trial is conducted in such a manner that the data collected do not permit the best possible information to be obtained, the subjects' expectations have been violated. Further, if poor research leads to a drug failing to be approved for marketing when in reality it is safe and efficacious, patients who would have benefited from the drug will be denied that opportunity.

The text of this volume contains no complicated statistical computation, and no complex statistical formulas are presented. Rather, the author addresses the issues conceptually and explains in an accessible and convincing manner that design, methodology, and analysis are of central and paramount importance in the research conducted by the pharmaceutical and biotechnology industries. The new drug development process requires the interdisciplinary collaboration of hundreds of clinical research professionals, and successful new drug development requires all of these individuals to conduct their part with full awareness of the personal responsibilities involved. The book's journey from drug discovery to post marketing surveillance is a fascinating one, and I believe that reading this book will prove informative to everyone involved with or interested in the process of new drug research and will enhance understanding of the importance of this work.

I strongly recommend this book to students of clinical research, pharmacy, and medicine and to all of my colleagues engaged in the wonderful and privileged field of developing new drugs that improve the human condition.

Jack Modell, M.D.
Global Vice President—Psychiatry
Neurosciences Medicines Development Center
GlaxoSmithKline

The views expressed are those of the writer individually, and not necessarily those of GlaxoSmithKline, his employer.

PREFACE

As indicated by the first part of its title, *New Drug Development*, this book provides an overview of the wide spectrum of activities involved in developing a new therapeutic drug. This spectrum starts with the initial stages of identifying a potentially useful drug candidate and concludes with the detailed monitoring of the drug's safety after it has been approved for marketing and is being prescribed for a large number of patients throughout the country. In between, it includes lead optimization, nonclinical and clinical evaluations of the drug's safety and efficacy profiles, and manufacturing considerations. The second part of the book's title, *Design, Methodology, and Analysis*, indicates the book's focus on the collection, analysis, and interpretation of numerical representations of information throughout this drug development process.

The book is written with two groups of readers in mind. The first is entry-level professionals in the pharmaceutical, biotechnology, and contract research organization industries and seasoned clinical research professionals who wish to refresh their knowledge in areas outside their immediate area of expertise. The second is students of clinical research, pharmacy, medicine, and allied health professions.

For the first audience, the book provides an introduction to new drug development and a core reference for discussions you will have with many members of study teams with whom you will work. These include professional statisticians and biomedical data scientists, clinical research associates, clinical monitors, clinical trial investigators, clinical trial administrators, managers, and coordinators, project managers, data managers, clinical scientists, regulatory affairs professionals, clinical operations specialists, medical writers, nurses, pharmacists, and medical safety officers. As well as becoming an expert at your own job, you will benefit greatly from being able to converse with all of these colleagues, and you will therefore become a much more valuable employee to your company.

For professors who may wish to consider using this book as a student textbook, several comments are appropriate. First, the book is the result of a course I teach in the Master of Science in Clinical Research degree program offered by Campbell University School of Pharmacy's Department of Clinical Research. Given the department's location in North Carolina's Research Triangle Park, next to world class pharmaceutical and biotechnology companies and contract research organizations, study design and analysis are discussed in the context of pharmaceutical clinical trials. The fourteen chapters fit well with this semester-long course. Second, the vast majority of references are books and book chapters, and these provide easily accessible sources of further information and resources for more detailed study. In addition, a list of Additional Resources for Training Executives and Professors is provided in the Appendix, indicating several books that may be particularly helpful as supplementary materials for lectures or may be designated as recommended additional reading for students. Third, PowerPoint slides for teaching support are available as detailed at the end of this preface.

Numerical information utilized in the drug development process takes many forms. Its collection and analysis vary from context to context, and its interpretation facilitates informed decision making. Study design and experimental methodology are concerned with the collection of optimum quality data, and analysis and interpretation are concerned with determining and interpreting the meaning of these data. Since the discipline of Statistics is concerned with design, methodology, and analysis, the book provides a conceptual introduction to Statistics and illustrates its important role in the new drug development process. For readers who may start to feel a little queasy at the very mention of the word "Statistics," please rest assured that this book is not a traditional statistics textbook. It does not present the detailed computational steps necessary to conduct an array of individual statistical tests. Rather, the book's chapters illustrate how the discipline of Statistics makes a central contribution to the complex process of new drug development by adopting a conceptual approach to the use of statistical analysis and the interpretation of the results obtained.

The defining goal of clinical research is to provide the evidence upon which evidence-based medicine is based. This evidence is typically provided to the clinical community in peer-reviewed clinical journal publications. A working knowledge of design, methodology, and analysis facilitates the ability to evaluate published results, distinguish well-conducted research from less well conducted research, and assess the relevance of high-quality research findings to the treatment of each individual patient.

Two comments on the book's contents are appropriate here. First, to improve the accessibility and flow of the book's material, the statistical concepts discussed are presented in a relatively pragmatic way. In many cases, I have resisted the temptation to say "Well, it is actually a bit more complicated or subtle than that." Such explication is better left in the hands of professional statisticians, and references are provided to excellent books by such professionals. Second, there is a certain degree of planned repetition in the book: Topics are introduced at one point and then integrated with other material at a later point. While unplanned repetition can be confusing, it is hoped that this planned strategy will be beneficial.

Throughout the presentation of the material in this book I have focused on two goals. One of them is to advocate the position that design, methodology, and analysis are central characters in the process of new drug development and that "statistics" are not simply obligatory and onerous "add-ons" at the end of research studies or simply abstractions for someone else to worry about. Rather, statistical awareness is an integral component that is constructively and meaningfully woven into the very fabric of new drug development. An awareness of design, methodology, and analysis is useful to everyone involved in this research, since such awareness reminds us of the supreme importance of acquiring optimum quality data throughout the process. The second goal is to emphasize that the ultimate purpose of new drug development is to produce a biologically active drug that is safe and that effectively treats biological states of clinical concern. In a very real sense, this is a book about biology.

Views expressed in this book are those of the author and Turner Medical Communications and not necessarily those of Campbell University and/or the Campbell University School of Pharmacy. I welcome comments on the book's text and suggestions for future improvements and can be contacted directly via my website, http://www.TurnerMedComm.com. Thank you for your interest in this book: I very much hope that you enjoy reading it.

PowerPoint slides based on this book are available for teaching support at the following Wiley FTP site: ftp://ftp.wiley.com/public/sci_tech_med/new_drug/.

J. Rick Turner
Chapel Hill, North Carolina
January 2007

ACKNOWLEDGMENTS

This format of this book evolved during several communications with Executive Editor Steve Quigley, and I gratefully acknowledge his initial input and continuing support throughout the project. I also thank Susanne Steitz, Jackie Palmieri, Fred Filler, Lisa Van Horn, and Marcia Felix at Wiley.

Throughout my careers in academe and the pharmaceutical industry, I have had the good fortune to work with some outstanding colleagues who are world leaders in their fields. I am very appreciative of the opportunities I have had to learn from these individuals and the friendships that we have developed.

I would like to acknowledge four particular influences on my thinking as it relates to this book. First, my undergraduate studies at the University of Sheffield provided a sound basis in experimental design and statistical analysis. Second, my understanding of, and appreciation for, the importance of study design in clinical trials has benefited considerably from reading the work of Steven Piantadosi, MD, PhD. Third, my awareness of the benefits of pharmacological therapy has been enhanced over the years by my mother's membership in the Royal Pharmaceutical Society of Great Britain and her more than fifty years of service as a community and hospital pharmacist. Fourth, I thank Rich Roberts for sharing his insights in molecular biology and his belief that knowledge of the structure of molecules is necessary to understand their function.

Several colleagues have provided assistance in the preparation of the book (responsibility for any inaccuracies remains mine alone). Alison Bowers, John Hewitt, and Wendy Stough reviewed initial drafts of various chapters and provided instructive feedback. Todd Durham reviewed the entire draft and provided insightful and extremely helpful comments that improved the final manuscript considerably, and I am very grateful for his contributions. The book was prepared in camera-ready format by Ms. Barrie Smith, President of The Perfect Page (see company web site http://www.theperfectpage.net). Artwork for this project was designed by Steve Shafer, Art Director at Shafer Productions, Inc. (see company web site http://www.ShaferProductions.com).

Deep appreciation for her love and support is expressed to my wife, Karen. Much companionship during the writing of this book was also provided by Misty and Mishadow, who spent many hours happily curled up on various leather chairs in my home office as I typed away late into the night.

Opening Quotes

Clinical trials should be designed, conducted, and analyzed according to sound scientific principles to achieve their objectives; and should be reported appropriately. The essence of rational drug development is to ask important questions and answer them with appropriate studies. The primary objectives of any study should be clear and explicitly stated.

ICH E8: General Considerations for Clinical Trials (1997)

Statistics is not only a discipline in its own right but it is also a fundamental tool for investigation in all biological and medical science.

Campbell and Machin (1999)

Biostatistics has been recognized and extensively employed as an indispensable tool for planning, conduct, and interpretation of clinical trials. In clinical research and development the biostatistician plays an important role that contributes toward the success of clinical trials. Well-prepared and open communication among clinicians, biostatisticians, and other related clinical research scientists will result in a successful clinical trial.

Chow and Liu (2004)

The most critical and difficult prerequisite for a good study is to select an important feasible question to answer. Accomplishing this is a consequence primarily of biological knowledge. Conceptual simplicity in design and analysis is a very important feature of good trials. Good trials are usually simple to analyze correctly.

Piantadosi (2005)

A statistically significant difference, no matter how small the P, does not mean that the difference is clinically important. A P value of <0.0001, if it emerges from a well-designed study, conveys a high degree of confidence that a difference really exists but says nothing about the magnitude of that difference or its clinical importance.

Fletcher and Fletcher (2005)

In recent years, a confluence of spectacular advances in chemistry, molecular biology, genomics, and chemical technology, and the cognate fields of spectroscopy, chromatography, and crystallography have led to the discovery and development of numerous novel therapeutic agents for the treatment of a wide spectrum of diseases.

Chorghade (2006)

PART I

INTRODUCTION

1

NEW DRUG DEVELOPMENT

1.1 INTRODUCTION

The term "drug" has various connotations in everyday language. In this book, it refers specifically to traditional pharmaceuticals and biopharmaceuticals that safely and effectively treat or prevent biological states of clinical concern. The text discusses the development of new ethical drugs, drugs that must be prescribed by a physician. The development of both small-molecule drugs and biopharmaceuticals is addressed. In the case of small-molecule drugs, attention focuses on the development of a drug containing a novel chemical compound, i.e., a new chemical entity (NCE) or new molecular entity (NME), as its active ingredient. In the case of biopharmaceuticals, attention focuses on proteins that are produced via the large-scale cultivation of microbial or mammalian cells.

New drug development is a lengthy, expensive, and complex endeavor. While precise quantification of "lengthy" and "expensive" is difficult, it is sufficient to note that respective values of 10–15 years and US$1,000,000,000 (one billion U.S. dollars) are realistic and informative approximations in 2007, the year of this book's publication. The complexity of this endeavor is well reflected in the observation that successful development and marketing approval of a new drug require the expertise and interdisciplinary cooperation of scientists and clinical researchers from many diverse disciplines. These include statistics, medicinal chemistry, molecular biology, bioinformatics and cheminformatics, pharmacology, pharmaceutical manufacturing, clinical trial operations, data collection and management, regulatory science, and medical writing, to name but a few.

The process of bringing a new drug from the research laboratory to marketing approval is not an easy journey, and the vast majority of new drugs that start the race will not make it to the finishing line. Again, precise quantification of the arduousness of this journey is difficult and unnecessary: The following reasonable estimates convey the message. For small-molecule drugs, only 10 out of 10,000 compounds discovered, synthesized, and screened make it to initial clinical trials in which the investigational drug is administered to humans for the first time. Of these 10, only one will successfully make it through all phases of clinical trials and be approved by a regulatory agency for marketing. The estimates for biotech drugs may have been different at one stage, but this situation may be changing. Meibohm (2006) noted that, compared with small-molecule drugs that entered the clinical phases of drug development between 1996 and 1998, biotech drugs that entered clinical trials during the same period had a fourfold greater chance of making it into the marketplace. However, Grabowski (2006) noted that the probability of success for biotech drugs is converging toward that for small-molecule drugs.

New Drug Development: Design, Methodology, and Analysis. By J. Rick Turner

1.2 ORIGIN AND GOALS OF THE BOOK

This book is the result of a course I teach in the Master of Science in Clinical Research degree program offered by the Department of Clinical Research in Campbell University's School of Pharmacy. In preparing this book I have attempted to follow the advice I give to students concerning the preparation of various types of regulatory documents and clinical publications: Be clear, concise, and contemporary. With regard to the latter of these desirable characteristics, the book includes discussions that capture contemporary trends in drug development and provides references to sources that address these topics in more detail. Over 60% of the references cited were published in 2004 or later. With regard to the first two characteristics, clarity and conciseness, judgment must be left to you.

One goal of this book is to provide a relatively brief and self-contained overview of new drug development, and a second is to illustrate the central role of the collection and analysis of numerical information in this process. Given the tremendous scale and complexity of new drug development, attempting to achieve these goals dictates that the contents need to be presented at an introductory level, and this is indeed the case. In this spirit, it is hoped that the book will be a useful road map for entry-level professionals in the pharmaceutical and biotechnology industries and in contract research organizations and for students interested in these areas of activity and potential employment.

1.3 THE DISCIPLINE OF STATISTICS

Throughout the book, statistical considerations are presented conceptually rather than computationally. It is hoped that, by the end of the book, the word "statistics" may appear less mysterious, irrelevant, or threatening to readers for whom the very mention of the word conjures up these or similar feelings.

For present purposes, the discipline of Statistics (recognized by the use of an upper case "S") can be thought of as encapsulating all of the considerations in the second part of the book's title, *Design, Methodology, and Analysis.* Statistics can be thought of as an integrated discipline that is important in all of the following activities:

- Identifying a research question that needs to be answered.
- Deciding upon the design of the study, the methodology that will be employed, and the numerical information (data) that will be collected.
- Presenting the design, methodology, and data to be collected in a study protocol. This study protocol specifies the manner of data collection and addresses all methodological considerations necessary to ensure the collection of optimum quality data for subsequent statistical analysis.

- Identifying the statistical techniques that will be used to describe and analyze the data in an associated statistical analysis plan, which should be written in conjunction with the study protocol.
- Describing and analyzing the data. This includes analyzing the variation in the data to see if there is compelling evidence that the drug is safe and effective. This process includes evaluation of the statistical significance of the results obtained and, very importantly, their clinical significance.
- Presenting the results of a clinical study to a regulatory agency in a clinical study report and presenting the results to the clinical community in journal publications.

There are several central tenets in this book. First, study design and statistical analysis are intimately and inextricably linked: The design of a study determines the analysis that will be used once the data have been collected. Second, experimental methodology is intimately related to both design and analysis. The goal of experimental methodology is to ensure that the data acquired during the study are of the highest possible quality. If this is not the case, the statistical analyses conducted on the data simply cannot produce the optimum quality information that leads to optimum quality interpretations. Third, quantitative information provides the rational basis for evidence-based decision making. Information is empowering. Evidence-based medicine (discussed in Chapter 13) is based on evidence collected during clinical research. The fourth tenet can be expressed as: Know where you are going when you start out, and plan accordingly at every stage of the journey. A shorter version of this sentiment is: Plan for success.

With regard to the phrase "plan for success," success is typically thought of in new drug development as obtaining approval from a regulatory agency to market the drug. However, it should be noted here that, due to the costs of pharmaceutical development, sometimes "success" can be thought of as identifying unsafe or ineffective products as soon as possible in a development program. (In this scenario, study design is just as critical.) Therefore, one might consider the overall goal of new product development as "Plan for success, but fail fast if failure is likely" (see Donahue and Ruberg, 1997).

When planning research studies in new drug development, two considerations are of critical importance. First, the statistical analyses that will eventually be conducted must be planned at the design stage of the study. Second, the desired goal, i.e., approval of a new drug by the appropriate regulatory agency, is known from the outset. Regulatory agencies provide enormous amounts of detailed guidance for the conduct and reporting of drug development research. This guidance should be studied before starting and borne in mind throughout the entire journey.

1.4 A LIFECYCLE PERSPECTIVE ON NEW DRUG DEVELOPMENT

The process of new drug development, as defined by bringing a new drug to marketing approval by a regulatory agency, can be represented by a three-stage model; drug discovery, nonclinical drug development, and clinical drug development. All of these stages are addressed in this book. However, two other areas of activity are crucial in the overall picture. One is manufacturing, addressed in Chapter 12. The other is postmarketing surveillance that occurs after regulatory marketing approval is granted. Postmarketing surveillance is introduced in Chapter 13 and discussed again in Chapter 14. Combined with discussions of drug discovery, nonclinical development, and clinical development, discussions of manufacturing and postmarketing surveillance allow the book to take a lifecycle perspective by following a new drug from inception to widespread use.

1.5 DESIGN, METHODOLOGY, AND ANALYSIS

The structural architecture for this book is presented schematically in Figure 1.1. This model comprises three components: design, methodology, and analysis. These components operate together in a process that is integrative, interactive, and ideally seamless. These components are three of the four central characters in this book: The fourth central character is identified in Section 1.11.

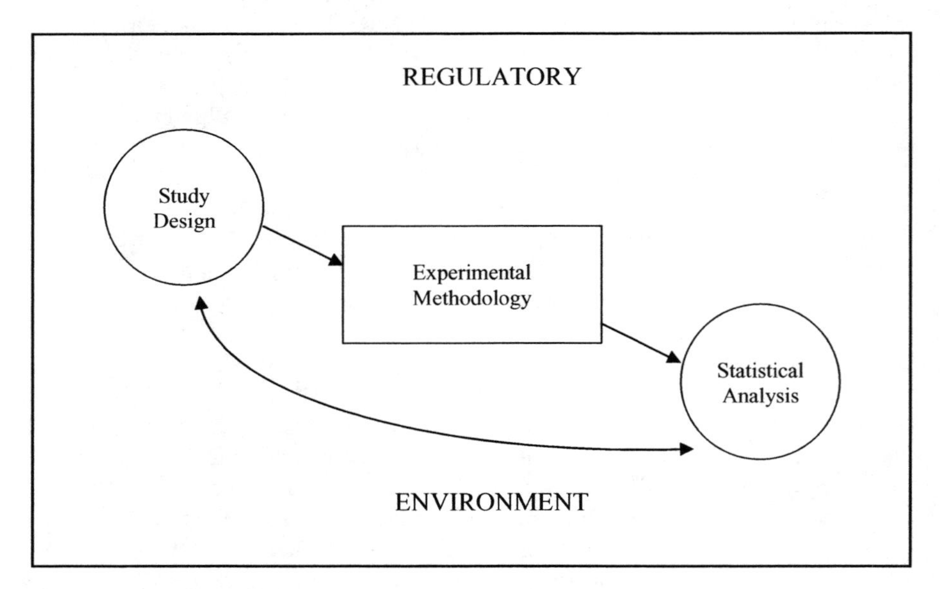

Figure 1.1. Design, methodology, and analysis in drug development.

1.5.1 The Term "Compelling Evidence"

Throughout this book the term "compelling evidence" is used when talking about the statistically significant results of statistical analyses. It is often said that the statistically significant results of a study "prove" something. The word prove is unfortunate in this context for various reasons. First, as will be seen in due course, a statistically significant result is a probabilistic statement, not an absolute statement. Second, the philosophy of scientific investigation makes it clear that it is not possible to prove a theory, only to disprove one (see Popper, 1935: reference provided to an English translation, 2002). As Popper commented, falsification is the criterion of demarcation between science and nonscience. Science is a process, a means of investigation. Individual sciences—e.g., physics, chemistry, biology—are scientific disciplines because they adopt the scientific method of inquiry. Theories lead to hypotheses, and these hypotheses are tested in the scientific manner. These hypotheses need to be able to be disproved. If repeated evaluations of a theory via appropriate hypothesis testing do not disprove it, compelling evidence starts to accumulate that the theory may have merit. It is then deemed reasonable to proceed on the basis that the theory does indeed have merit, with the knowledge and acceptance that future investigations may provide evidence that the theory is in fact false.

1.6 DRUG DISCOVERY

Drug discovery can be thought of as the work done from the time of the identification of a therapeutic need in a particular disease area to the time the drug candidate deemed most likely to safely affect the desired therapeutic benefit is identified. This drug candidate may be a small molecule or a biological macromolecule such as a protein or nucleic acid. Drug discovery activities vary between small molecules and biological macromolecules, but, once a drug candidate has been identified and moves into the drug development phase, the regulatory governance of nonclinical and clinical research and the marketing approval process is very similar in both cases.

1.7 NONCLINICAL DEVELOPMENT

Before discussing nonclinical development, it is worth noting that discussions about the use of the nomenclature "nonclinical" versus "preclinical" are not infrequent and are sometimes heated. Nonhuman animal research is currently necessary before regulatory permission will be given to test a new drug in humans. Since part of the overall nonhuman animal testing is done before the drug is first given to humans, the term preclinical has a certain appeal. However, a significant amount of nonhuman animal testing is typically conducted after the first administration of the drug to humans. Some of the more lengthy, more complex, and more expensive nonhuman animal testing is typically not started until initial human testing reveals that the drug has a good safety profile in humans and therefore has a reasonable chance of being approved for marketing if it also proves to be effective in later clinical trials. In this book, the term nonclinical has been adopted for research involving nonhuman animals.

Once selected, the drug candidate moves to nonclinical development. While human pharmacological therapy is the ultimate goal, understanding nonclinical drug safety and efficacy is critical to subsequent rationally designed, ethical human trials. The term "efficacy" is used in drug development to refer to the desired therapeutic (biological) effect of the candidate drug. Nonclinical research involves both *in vitro* and *in vivo* testing, and gathers critical information concerning drug dose, frequency, and route of administration.

1.8 CLINICAL DEVELOPMENT

Clinical trials examine the safety and efficacy of interventions, or treatments, in human subjects. This book focuses on pharmaceutical clinical trials. The word "subject" is used deliberately here, since all participants in clinical trials are subjects, even if they are under the care of a personal physician, and therefore patients in that context, at the time of the trial. The key difference between clinical care and clinical research is that clinical research is conducted for the general good of the population at large, not for the specific individual benefit of the participants in the study, while clinical care is concerned with the specific well-being of each individual patient.

Once clinical research studies are completed and a drug has been approved for marketing by a regulatory agency, reports of the drug's safety and efficacy will be published in the clinical literature. This dissemination of the results provides clinicians and research scientists with evidence of the beneficial administration of the drug. This information can then be considered by clinicians for use in the practice of evidence-based medicine, i.e., clinical care predicated on the available evidence and then specifically tailored to the unique needs of each individual patient. Patients thus benefit from the knowledge gained in a clinical trial when their clinicians read medical journal articles describing the benefits of a certain treatment and decide that the treatment would be beneficial for them.

It is worth noting here that a participant in a clinical trial, i.e., a subject in our nomenclature, may benefit from the drug being tested once it has been approved. At that time, the participant is now a patient and will benefit from a trial in which he or she participated. However, when actually involved in the trial, the patient was engaging in clinical research as a subject.

Pharmaceutical and biotechnology companies often use contract research organizations (CROs) to conduct clinical trials for them. These are specialist companies that conduct clinical research for many companies (see Nichol, 2006). Contract manufacturing organizations (CMOs) are also used by many companies. In this context, the term "sponsor" is frequently used to refer to a company that has contracted a CRO to conduct a trial or a CMO to manufacture a drug.

1.8.1 Ethical Conduct

Treating subjects in clinical trials in an ethical manner is of paramount importance. Several fundamental ethical principles guide drug development research in clinical trials, including:

- Clinical equipoise. Clinical equipoise exists when all of the available evidence about a new drug does not show that it is more beneficial than an alternative and, equally, does not show that it is less beneficial than the alternative. For example, to be able to conduct a clinical trial that involves administering an investigational drug to some individuals and a control treatment (often a placebo) to others, there cannot be any evidence that suggests that the investigational drug shows greater efficacy than the control treatment or that it leads to greater side effects than the control treatment. When individuals agree to participate in a clinical trial, they do so with the understanding that all of the treatments in the trial are assumed to be of equal value. By the end of the trial, there may be compelling evidence that the investigational drug is safe and more effective than the control treatment, but the trial must be started with a good faith belief that the drug and the control treatment are of equal merit.
- Respect for persons. This principle necessitates that investigators give potential participants all pertinent information about the study and answer any questions. If a potential participant then agrees to participate voluntarily (i.e., he or she is not coerced in any real or implied manner), informed consent is obtained. This involves obtaining the subject's written permission (or the written permission of a parent or guardian) to participate in the study. It also necessitates protecting potential subjects with possibly impaired decision-making capacity and maintaining confidentiality of all information obtained at every stage of the study procedures.
- Beneficence. This principle requires that the study design is scientifically sound and that any risks of the research are acceptable in relation to the likely benefits from the study (in terms of knowledge obtained that will likely benefit a large number of individuals).
- Justice. This principle requires that the burdens and benefits of participation in clinical trials are distributed evenly and fairly. Historically, populations that were easily and conveniently accessed by researchers, such as prison inmates, nursing home residents, and people with poor access to general health care, have been used when they should not have been. Vulnerable populations should not be deliberately chosen for participation in clinical trials when nonvulnerable populations would also be appropriate. The benefits of

participation, such as access to potentially life-saving new therapies, should be available to all, including those not historically well represented such as women, children, and members of ethnic minorities.

Derenzo and Moss (2006) captured the importance of ethical considerations in all aspects of clinical studies in the following quote:

> Each study component has an ethical aspect. The ethical aspects of a clinical trial cannot be separated from the scientific objectives. Segregation of ethical issues from the full range of study design components demonstrates a flaw in understanding the fundamental nature of research involving human subjects. Compartmentalization of ethical issues is inconsistent with a well-run trial. Ethical and scientific considerations are intertwined (p. 4).

Ethical considerations are of the utmost importance in clinical research, and the ethical aspects of new drug development will be highlighted throughout this book. (See also Salek and Edgar, 2002.)

1.8.2 Different Studies in Clinical Development

While the efficacy of an approved drug is extremely relevant, so too is its safety profile, sometimes referred to as its toxicity profile since every drug will have some unwanted side effects. Initial safety evaluations are conducted in healthy adult subjects in first time in human (FTIH) studies. The terms "healthy volunteers" or "normal volunteers" are often seen in this context, but they seem particularly unsuitable: By definition, all participants in all clinical trials are volunteers, and the use of the word "volunteer" in just FTIH trials could mistakenly be seen to imply that participants in other trials are not volunteers. Additionally, the word "normal" seems questionable in that it may mistakenly be seen to imply that subjects in other trials are abnormal in ways not related to having or not having the disease or condition of interest. The term "healthy adult subjects" circumvents such misperceptions.

If all goes well in FTIH trials, the investigative drug is administered to relatively small numbers of subjects with the medical disease or condition of relevance. If all goes well in these trials, larger trials in which the investigative drug is administered to a much larger number of subjects with the disease or condition of relevance are conducted. The goal of these trials is to provide statistically significant and clinically significant evidence of the drug product's efficacy and to provide further evidence of its safety and tolerability (the terms "statistically significant" and "clinically significant" are discussed in detail in Chapter 7 and Chapter 8, respectively). These larger trials are undertaken towards the end of a drug development program with the goal of providing an answer to a specific research question concerning the efficacy of the drug product. The data collected in these trials are very important in facilitating a regulatory agency's deliberations concerning the possible approval of the drug for marketing.

After a drug is approved for marketing, additional data are collected. These focus on its safety and its effectiveness. The term "effectiveness" can be meaningfully distinguished from the term efficacy. Efficacy is evaluated during tightly controlled clinical trials in which on the order of 3,000–5,000 subjects participate. While this may seem a large number at first, once the drug is marketed, it may be prescribed to hundreds of thousands of patients. These patients will comprise a much more diverse set of individuals than the set of people who took part in the clinical trials, and they will likely take the drug in a less controlled (more realistic) manner. This occurrence has two implications. First, rare side effects may surface, and these need to be identified and investigated: Rare adverse reactions are probabilistically unlikely to be seen in a clinical trial, even though it may have several thousand participants. Second, the therapeutic benefit of the drug in this larger context, i.e., its effectiveness, needs to be evaluated.

Therefore, postmarketing surveillance is conducted to examine safety and effectiveness. The terms "pharmacovigilance" and "pharmacosurveillance" studies are also used in this context. Pharmacosurveillance monitors all reports of adverse reactions and thus compiles extended safety data. Pharmacosurveillance is therefore a critical component of the overall process of ensuring all members of a target disease population receive the greatest protection from adverse reactions.

1.9 PHARMACEUTICAL MANUFACTURING

Pharmaceutical and biopharmaceutical manufacturing is also an essential consideration in the process of new drug development. When the drug candidate has been identified in drug discovery, it must be administered in nonclinical trials and then in clinical trials. The drug product has to be administered in a certain form in clinical trials, such as a tablet or an injection. Manufacturing the tablet or injection is an extremely complex procedure. Moreover, if the drug molecule of interest cannot be successfully administered, and eventually successfully manufactured and placed on the market in a suitable form (one that can be readily transported from the manufacturing plant to the pharmacy and one that has a suitable and stable shelf-life), it is not useful for widespread clinical practice no matter how potentially beneficial it may be.

Manufacturing processes differ according to the stage of new drug development. Initially, very small amounts of the drug are needed, and typically made on a laboratory scale. This amount becomes progressively larger as the clinical development program proceeds. Eventually, marketing of the drug requires full-scale commercial manufacturing. Moving from small-scale production via pilot manufacturing plants to commercial manufacturing plants is far more complex than simply building proportionately larger manufacturing equipment. Manufacturing considerations are addressed in Chapter 12.

1.10 DEFINITIONS OF CLINICAL RESEARCH AND CLINICAL TRIALS

Since the terms "clinical research" and "clinical trial" occur many times in this book, it is appropriate to provide some helpful definitions at this time.

1.10.1 Clinical Research

Clinical research is a very wide field of investigation and one whose breadth and complexity has attracted various definitions. The National Institutes of Health (NIH) provided this definition on its web site (http://www.nih.gov):

> NIH defines human clinical research as: **(1)** Patient-oriented research. Research conducted with human subjects (or on material of human origin such as tissues, specimens and cognitive phenomena) for which an investigator (or colleague) directly interacts with human subjects. Excluded from this definition are *in vitro* studies that utilize human tissues that cannot be linked to a living individual. Patient-oriented research includes: (a) mechanisms of human disease, (b) therapeutic interventions, (c) clinical trials, or (d) development of new technologies. **(2)** Epidemiologic and behavioral studies. **(3)** Outcomes research and health services research.

Throughout the edited volume entitled *Principles and Practice of Clinical Research,* Gallin (2002a) and contributors adopted the definition of the Association of American Medical Colleges Task Force on Clinical Research. As cited by Gallin (2002b), this task force defined clinical research as:

> A component of medical and health research intended to produce knowledge essential for understanding human disease, preventing and treating illness, and promoting health. Clinical research embraces a continuum of studies involving interaction with patients, diagnostic clinical materials or data, or populations, in any of these categories: disease mechanisms; translational research; clinical knowledge; detection, diagnosis and natural history of disease; therapeutic interventions including clinical trials; prevention and health promotion; behavioral research; health services research; epidemiology; and community-based and managed care-based research (p. 1).

In their volume entitled *Translational and Experimental Clinical Research* (Schuster and Powers, 2005), a more succinct definition was provided by Schuster (2005):

> Clinical research includes any scientific investigation in which the unit of analysis is the person. If n is the number of human beings from which the information is derived, the study can legitimately be characterized as clinical research (p. xvii).

As Schuster noted, this definition is "simple, practical, and unambiguous," and it is helpful for discussions throughout this book.

1.10.2 Clinical Trials

The National Institutes of Health defined a clinical trial on its web site (http://www.nih.gov, accessed September 14, 2006) as:

> A prospective biomedical or behavioral research study of human subjects that is designed to answer specific questions about biomedical or behavioral interventions (drugs, treatments, devices, or new ways of using known drugs, treatments, or devices).

Piantadosi (2005) provided a more succinct definition:

> A clinical trial is an experiment testing a medical treatment on human subjects (p. 16).

1.10.3 Drug Clinical Trials

Pharmaceutical and biopharmaceutical clinical trials fall within the domain of clinical research as provided by these descriptions. The primary focus of this book concerns clinical trials conducted during the development of new drugs, one of the categories in this definition (see Becker and Whyte, 2006, for discussions of clinical trials for medical devices and Piantadosi, 2005, for discussion of clinical trials for surgical procedures).

1.11 THE FOURTH CENTRAL CHARACTER IN THIS BOOK—BIOLOGY

The statement that this is a book about biology may seem strange, especially given that words like "design," "methodology," "analysis," and "Statistics" have been encountered already, and are pervasive throughout the following chapters. However, the word "clinical" in the terms "clinical research" and "clinical trials" points us in the direction of biology and the biological significance of a drug's effects.

Clinical research and clinical trials investigate topics of clinical relevance, and, in the context of this book, clinical relevance is intimately related to biological relevance. The ultimate goal of new drug development is to produce a biologically active drug that is reasonably safe, well tolerated, and useful in the treatment or prevention of patients' biological states that are of clinical concern. (The word "reasonably" in the previous sentence may initially seem strange, but, as noted in Section 1.8.2, all drugs have some side effects. The important goal, therefore, is to ensure a reasonable benefit/risk ratio: This will be discussed further later in the book.) The engine that drives new drug development is an unmet medical need, which is ultimately an unmet biological need.

Drug discovery and design focuses on the identification of compounds that are potentially biologically active, and the optimization of lead candidate drug molecules focuses on maximizing the probability of biological activity while also maximizing the drug molecule's safety. Topics such as the drug's progress through the body toward its target receptor (a biological structure), drug-receptor interaction and the resulting generation of a biological signal, metabolic pathways, biomarkers, genetics and bioinformatics, and measuring biological changes following drug administration (either via clinical endpoints or surrogate endpoints) indicate the extent of biological considerations in drug development. All of these topics are discussed at various points in the following chapters.

Piantadosi (2005) made the following observation about clinical trials and the need for experimental design, experimental methodology, and statistical analysis:

> Experimental design and analysis have become essential because of the greater detail in modern biological theories and the complexities in treatments of disease. The clinician is usually interested in small, but biologically important, treatment effects that can be obscured by uncontrolled natural variation and bias in non-rigorous studies. This places well-performed clinical trials at the very center of clinical research today (pp. 9-10).

Campbell and Machin (1999) also commented about the role of Statistics in biological investigations:

> Statistics is not only a discipline in its own right but it is also a fundamental tool for investigation in all biological and medical science. As such, any serious investigator in these fields must have a grasp of the basic principles. With modern computer facilities there is little need for familiarity with the technical details of statistical calculations. However, a physician should understand when such calculations are valid, when they are not, and how they should be interpreted.

This book, which focuses on biological considerations in clinical trials, is written very much in this spirit. While study design, experimental methodology, and statistical analysis are central characters in our discussions of new drug development, their importance lies in their role in the development of drugs that influence a patient's biology for the better.

2

THE REGULATORY ENVIRONMENT FOR NEW DRUG DEVELOPMENT

2.1 INTRODUCTION

This chapter introduces the regulatory environment in which new drug development is conducted. The current regulatory environment is largely a result of the work of the International Conference on Harmonisation (ICH) of Technical Requirements for Registration of Pharmaceuticals for Human Use. The ICH is an amalgamation of expertise from various agencies and organizations across the world.

The ICH arose since the regulations for submitting documentation requesting marketing approval of a drug were historically quite different between countries. Data requirements around the world were dissimilar, meaning that studies often had to be repeated to satisfy national regulatory requirements if marketing permission was desired in multiple countries. This lack of uniformity meant that nonhuman animal (nonclinical) and human (clinical) studies had to be repeated, resulting in additional and unnecessary use of animal, human, and material resources. It also meant that bringing a drug to market in various countries took longer than necessary, delaying its availability to patients.

Harmonization of regulatory requirements was pioneered by the European Community (now the European Union) in the 1980s, as it moved towards the development of a single market for pharmaceuticals. The success achieved in Europe demonstrated that harmonization was feasible. The harmonization process was then extended to include Japan and the United States. The ICH was formed from a government body and an industry association from each of these regions. These bodies and associations as listed by Molzon (2006) are:

- The European Commission and the European Federation of Pharmaceutical Industries and Associations (The European Agency for the Evaluation of Medicines is also a party to the ICH).
- The Japanese Ministry of Health, Labour and Welfare, and the Japan Pharmaceutical Manufacturers Association.
- The United States Food and Drug Administration (specifically, the Center for Drug Evaluation and Research and the Center for Biologics Evaluation and Research), and the Pharmaceutical Research and Manufacturers of America.

b*New Drug Development: Design, Methodology, and Analysis.* By J. Rick Turner

2.1.1 Goals of the ICH

The ICH has several goals, including:

- To maintain a forum for a constructive dialog between regulatory authorities and the pharmaceutical industry on differences in technical requirements for marketing approval in the European Union, the United States, and Japan in order to ensure a more timely introduction of new drugs and hence their availability to patients.
- To facilitate the adoption of new or improved technical research and development approaches that update or replace current practices. These new or improved practices should permit a more economical use of animal, human, and material resources without compromising safety.
- To monitor and update harmonized technical requirements leading to a greater mutual acceptance of research and development data.
- To contribute to the protection of public health from an international perspective.
- To encourage the implementation and integration of common standards of documentation and submission of regulatory applications by disseminating harmonized guidelines.

To facilitate the last goal, the ICH has produced many guidance documents for sponsors to use in various aspects of drug development research and documentation, including drug safety, efficacy, and quality. Some of these that apply to design, methodology, and statistical considerations are specifically cited in following chapters. Readers are referred to the ICH web site for more detailed information (http://www.ich.org).

2.2 THE FOOD AND DRUG ADMINISTRATION

Since there are many regulatory agencies throughout the world, I have respectfully used the general phrase "regulatory agency" wherever possible in this book rather than singling out a particular one. However, since I live and work in the United States, specific reference to its regulatory agency does occur at times.

The United States government has three branches (executive, legislative, and judicial), and several agencies are part of the executive branch, which is charged with carrying out the statutory laws created by the legislative branch. Agencies therefore create regulations or administrative law (RAPS, 2005). The regulatory agency responsible for the governance of new drug development in the United States is the Food and Drug Administration (FDA).

The FDA is housed within the Public Health Service, part of the Department of Health and Human Services. Redefined in the 1997 FDA Modernization Act, the

FDA's relatively broad mission includes providing reasonable assurances that foods and cosmetics (both of which are regulated products) are safe and that drugs and devices (also regulated products) are safe and effective. Several program centers facilitate the FDA's operations, including:

- The Center for Drug Evaluation and Research (CDER).
- The Center for Biologics Evaluation and Research (CBER).
- The Center for Veterinary Medicine (CVM).
- The Center for Devices and Radiological Health (CDRH).
- The Center for Food Safety and Applied Nutrition (CFSAN).

To accomplish its mission, the FDA's internal structure includes the Office of Regulatory Affairs, which is responsible for ensuring that regulated products comply with public health laws and regulations. Within this office are the Office of Enforcement and the Office of Criminal Investigations. The FDA is therefore a law enforcement agency. To carry out such enforcement, it has both administrative and judicial means at its disposal. It typically attempts to achieve compliance with its statutes using administrative means, such as inspections of products and manufacturing facilities, notices of violation of regulations, recalls (voluntary and mandatory) of regulated products from the marketplace, and (adverse) publicity. Should these administrative means fail to achieve compliance, however, the FDA can utilize the U.S. court system and the Department of Justice's assistance to invoke its judicial tools, which include seizure, injunction, and prosecution (RAPS, 2005). If FDA agents appear at your place of employment with serious expressions and carrying an official-looking document and side-arms, it may be judicious to call your company's legal advisors. Companies have compliance departments to provide advice and internal audits and hopefully prevent this occurrence.

The FDA becomes involved in new drug development when nonclinical research conducted by a sponsor starts to indicate that the investigative drug has potential benefits in humans (Ascione, 2001). Regulatory oversight does not apply to drug discovery and design, and some of the earlier aspects of nonclinical development are not conducted under regulatory oversight either. However, many later aspects of nonclinical development and all aspects of clinical development are conducted under regulatory governance. This governance also includes manufacturing processes.

2.2.1 The Code of Federal Regulations

The *Federal Register* is a collection of substantive regulations that is published by the government every weekday with the exception of federal holidays. The *Code of Federal Regulations* (CFR), which is revised annually, is a codification of the general and permanent rules published in the *Federal Register*. It is divided into

50 titles, each of which is further divided into subchapters, parts, subparts, and sections. The FDA regulations are in Title 21 of the CFR, commonly referred to as "21 CFR." Individual regulations have more detailed identifiers; 21 CFR 310.3, for example, provides the code's definition of a new drug. (See Bowers, 2005, for additional discussion.)

2.3 cGMP, cGLP, AND cGCP

These three acronyms are very common in literature pertaining to new drug development. They refer to good manufacturing practice (GMP), good laboratory practice (GLP), and good clinical practice (GCP). The various stages of new drug development should be conducted according to the appropriate regulations and guidances. The initial "c" in each case stands for the word "current." The implication here is that, in the years between rewrites of regulations and guidances, certain modifications in the generally accepted best way of performing a certain activity (best practices) may occur. Therefore, while the guidance as written in the most recent version reflects the "official" stance, it is considered wise to conform to the modified ideology as appropriate.

2.4 REGULATORY ASPECTS OF NEW DRUG DEVELOPMENT

There are many regulatory requirements for new drug development and approval. Before a sponsor submits a request for a drug to be registered for human use, a tremendous amount of highly specified laboratory testing, nonclinical work, and clinical trials need to be performed. In all cases, the procedures and results must be documented appropriately. From a regulatory perspective, if the research is not documented, for all intents and purposes, it has not been done.

This applies to nonclinical development as well as clinical development. Nonclinical work is reported to the FDA in an Investigational New Drug Application (IND). This document is reviewed to see if clinical work should be allowed to start. Once the clinical development program is completed, all of the developmental work will be reported to the FDA in a New Drug Application (NDA) or a Biologicals License Application (BLA). If the review of these enormous documents goes well, the drug will be approved for marketing.

The new drug development and approval process includes several principal steps (RAPS, 2005):

- Nonclinical testing.
- Submission of an IND.
- FDA review of the IND.
- Preparation and submission of an NDA or a BLA following clinical research.
- FDA review and approval of the NDA or BLA.

While this list of items is a useful and succinct description of the fundamental steps in achieving marketing approval for a new drug, such approval represents the culmination of many years of complex research conducted by many people at a cost of many millions of dollars. The highly abbreviated descriptions in the following sections of this chapter cannot begin to address the full complexities of the regulatory environment. Rather, they are intended to serve as an indicator of the tremendous importance of the regulatory environment and as a high-level road map for your further study of this area.

2.5 SPONSOR AND REGULATORY AGENCY RESPONSIBILITIES

Hagglof and Holmgren (2006) summarized the roles and responsibilities of the sponsor and the regulatory agency for drug products. Marketing approval of a drug is a contract between the sponsor and the regulatory agency, and the conditions of the approval are spelled out in detail and also condensed in the prescribing information. Any planned changes on the part of the sponsor need to be presented to the agency, and new approval is necessary in many cases. The regulatory agency's roles and responsibilities include:

- Approving the clinical trial application.
- Approving drugs that have been scientifically evaluated to provide evidence of a satisfactory benefit/risk ratio (the balance between the therapeutic advantages of receiving the drug and possible risks).
- Monitoring the safety of the marketed drug.
- In serious cases, withdrawing the license for marketing. This can occur for various reasons, including failure of adequate additional information being included in the prescribing information after adverse reactions are reported and failure to be compliant with regulations concerning drug manufacture.

The sponsor's roles and responsibilities include:

- Keeping all pertinent documentation related to the drug up to date and ensuring it complies with standards set by the current state of scientific knowledge and the regulatory agency.
- Collecting, compiling, and evaluating safety data and submitting regular reports to the regulatory agency.
- Taking rapid action where necessary. This includes withdrawal of a particular batch of the drug or withdrawal of the entire product if warranted.

The relevance and importance of the regulatory environment cannot be overemphasized. This overview of the roles and responsibilities of both the sponsor and the regulatory agency serves to illustrate the interaction between the two, both before and after a drug is approved for marketing. As well as being experts on current regulations, Regulatory Affairs professionals keep in constant dialog with regulatory agencies throughout the drug development process.

2.6 THE INVESTIGATIONAL NEW DRUG APPLICATION

If all has gone well in a nonclinical development program, a sponsor submits an IND (the acronym for Investigational New Drug Application does not include an "A"). The term investigational new drug describes an unapproved drug that is to be used in clinical trials. The IND is the means through which a sponsor advances to its clinical development program.

An IND is actually a request for an exemption from a particular federal statute. Current federal law requires that a drug has been approved for marketing before it can be transported or distributed across state lines. Therefore, officially, an investigational new drug cannot be shipped across state lines in interstate commerce because, by definition, it has not been approved for marketing. Given the predominance of multicenter clinical trials in drug development (particularly in the later-stage clinical trials), a sponsor will very likely want to ship the investigational new drug to clinical investigators in many states. The sponsor therefore has to request an exemption from statute prohibiting this. The IND is the means through which the sponsor technically obtains this exemption from the FDA.

The regulations pertaining to INDs are located in 21 CFR 312 and provide detailed guidance for both content and format. Interestingly, a sponsor does not hear from the FDA if the FDA's review is positive. The FDA reviewers have 30 days to respond to the sponsor following submission of the IND. If the sponsor has not been contacted in that window, they have implied permission to commence the clinical development program described in the IND.

In scientific terms, the purpose of an IND is to provide detailed documentation that will allow the FDA to conclude that it is reasonable for the sponsor to proceed to clinical trials. Generally, this includes data and information in four broad areas:

- Animal pharmacology and toxicology studies. These nonclinical data permit an assessment of whether the product is considered to be reasonably safe for initial testing in humans. The phrase "considered to be reasonably safe" may sound somewhat less than definitive or reassuring, but it is simply the case that no amount of nonclinical testing can guarantee that a drug will be absolutely safe when administered to humans (see Section 4.5). As in many instances in the new drug development process, an informed judgment has to be made, on this occasion by the regulatory agency (see Section 14.5.1).
- Manufacturing information. These data address the composition, manufacture, stability, and controls used for manufacturing the drug. This information is provided to document the sponsor's ability to produce and supply consistent batches of high-quality drug.

- Clinical study protocols. Protocols include precise accounts of the design, methodology, and analysis considerations necessary to conduct the proposed studies and analyze their results (see Section 5.7). Therefore, design, methodology, and analysis information must be submitted in study protocol format before administering the investigational new drug to the first human subject. These detailed protocols for the proposed initial-phase clinical studies are provided to allow the FDA to assess whether the trials will expose subjects to unnecessary risks.
- Investigator information. Information on the qualifications of clinical investigators is provided to allow assessment of whether they are qualified to fulfill their duties at the investigational sites used during the clinical trials.

2.6.1 Review of the Investigational New Drug Application

When submitting an IND, a sponsor should state the goals that make up the overall clinical development program. When originally submitted, the general investigational plan should outline the overall plan, but it only need articulate the studies to be conducted during the first year of clinical development. Subsequent IND updates provide additional details. The FDA's overall review process consists of several reviews, including medical/clinical, chemistry, pharmacology/toxicology, and statistical (see Dubey et al., 2006, for more details).

The medical/clinical review.

This review is conducted by medical officers who are almost always physicians. Medical reviewers are responsible for evaluating the safety of the clinical protocols in an IND. Typically, a company will open an IND with a single study and then add new study protocols over time. Protocols are reviewed to determine if the subjects will be protected from unnecessary risks and if the respective study designs will provide data relevant to evaluating the safety and efficacy of the drug. Under federal regulations, proposed Phase I trials are evaluated almost exclusively for safety considerations. The initial IND is amended and updated over time to add new study protocols, submit reports of completed studies, and keep the FDA informed of all the data that the company is gathering on the investigational drug. When evaluating study protocols for Phase II and Phase III trials, the reviewers also must ensure that these studies are of sufficient scientific quality to be capable of providing data that can support marketing approval (see Section 10.2 for discussion of the nature of Phase I, II, and III clinical trials).

The chemistry review.

Chemists are responsible for reviewing the chemistry and manufacturing control (CMC) sections of the IND. These sections address issues related to drug identity, manufacturing control, and analysis. Drug manufacturing and processing procedures need to ensure that the compound is stable and can be consistently made to high standards. The IND should describe any chemistry and manufacturing differences between the nature of the investigational drug proposed for clinical use and the drug product that was used in the animal toxicology trials that formed the basis for the sponsor's conclusion that it was safe to proceed to clinical studies. If there are any such differences, the sponsor should discuss if and how these differences might affect the safety profile of the clinical drug product.

The pharmacology/toxicology review.

This review is conducted by pharmacologists and toxicologists who evaluate the results of animal testing and attempt to relate animal drug effects to potential drug effects in humans. The IND should provide a description of the pharmacological effects and the mechanism(s) of action of the drug in animals (if known) and information on the pharmacokinetics (absorption, distribution, metabolism, and excretion) of the drug. An integrated summary of the toxicological effects of the drug *in vitro* and in animals is also required. (In cases where species specificity or other considerations make many or all animal toxicological models irrelevant, the sponsor is encouraged to contact the agency to discuss toxicological testing.)

The statistical review.

The CDER has several offices, including the Office of Pharmacoepidemiology and Statistical Science. This office contains the Office of Biostatistics. One of the Office of Biostatistics' responsibilities is to develop statistical and mathematical methods to enhance the drug review process in various areas, including:

- Pharmacokinetics and pharmacodynamics.
- Bioavailability and bioequivalence.
- Drug safety monitoring.
- Demonstration of efficacy.
- Chemical testing and product quality assessment and control.

The Office of Biostatistics has taken the lead in the development of several guidance documents on specific topics, including ICH E9, Statistical Principles in Clinical Trials, and ICH E10, Choice of Control Groups in Clinical Trials. It is advisable for sponsors to follow these guidances.

In the IND statistical review, study protocols are reviewed somewhat differently according to the phase of the proposed study. Phase I study protocols, which are evaluated for safety, may not receive a statistical review. Study protocols for studies in which efficacy is evaluated and the results of which are intended to be used as supportive evidence of efficacy will likely receive a statistical review. This may be particularly likely if the study includes a large sample size. Most Phase III trials receive a statistical review. Since Phase III trials are undertaken to provide compelling evidence of both safety and efficacy, all of the design, methodology, and analysis considerations need to be addressed satisfactorily, making many aspects of the protocol of interest to the statistical reviews. Questions of interest to the statisticians include:

- Does the design facilitate collection of data that are appropriate for addressing the study objectives and reduce the potential for bias?
- Are the primary endpoints relevant?
- Have the criteria that will be used to determine efficacy been precisely specified?
- Have the randomization schedule and all aspects of methodology (operational and measurement) been detailed adequately?
- Have sample-size estimates been conducted appropriately and is the study powered as needed?
- Has adequate statistical care been taken in analytical strategies dealing with repeated measurements and with missing data?
- Are the planned analytical strategies appropriate for the design and capable of providing answers?

The statistical review may also take a more global view and, in addition to evaluating the aspects of each protocol in a stand-alone fashion, evaluate how it fits in with and adds to the overall drug development program.

Following initial clearance of an IND (INDs are never formally "approved") and throughout the time that the studies included in it are being conducted, the IND application must be updated continuously. In addition to annual reports, protocol amendments must be submitted any time that a protocol is changed or if the sponsor wishes to use a new study protocol. Study reports of completed trials are also submitted so that documentation is submitted as it becomes available. This "build as you go" concept is central to the IND philosophy, and a company should not withhold information about an investigational product from the FDA.

2.7 THE NEW DRUG APPLICATION

At the completion of the clinical trials conducted using an investigational new drug, and the completion of all nonclinical studies being conducted contemporaneously, a New Drug Application (NDA: this time the acronym does include an "A") is filed. The regulations pertaining to NDAs are located in 21 CFR 314 and, as for INDs, provide detailed guidance for both content and format.

Typically, sponsors meet with the FDA to discuss the content and format of an NDA prior to its preparation. Such a "pre-NDA meeting" can be crucial for the sponsor to understand the content and format that will best facilitate the review process for a given submission.

Historically, NDAs, like other regulatory documents, were submitted on paper, and the total amount of paperwork was enormous. A typical paper NDA submission might constitute 400 volumes, each 400 pages long. The process is now moving toward electronic submission, which has many advantages, including the fact that hyperlinks can be incorporated that allow a reviewer to navigate directly from one part of the submission to another. This is particularly valuable for statistical reviewers who may wish to navigate from the Methods section of a clinical study report to tabulated data presented in the Results section and then to the supporting raw data sets.

2.7.1 Statistical Review of the New Drug Application

The comments here focus on the statistical review of the NDA. The major difference between an IND and an NDA submission is that, when the NDA is submitted, the studies proposed in the IND have been conducted, and analysis and interpretation of the data collected are included. The FDA's review of the NDA focuses on determining if it finds the evidence concerning safety, efficacy, and manufacturing ability to be compelling and if it is therefore prepared to approve the drug for marketing. The FDA's statistical reviewers play a major role in making this determination. Statistical reviewers typically review both the Statistics and Clinical Data sections, and they are also available to review other sections.

The statisticians conducting the review of an NDA evaluate the statistical relevance of the data presented so that they can provide the medical officers with information concerning how well the findings are likely to generalize to the larger patient population in the country. They evaluate the extent of any deviations from the protocols submitted in the IND in the conduct of the study as well as the overall quality of the data collected. All clinical study protocol amendments are reviewed to see what deviations from the original study design have occurred and how these (and deviations that were not detailed in protocol amendments) may have influenced the data.

Having access to all study data in electronic form allows the FDA's statisticians to replicate all analyses that are reported, and, importantly, to conduct any alternative and additional analyses they feel are warranted and which may help them to reach an informed decision concerning recommendation of the drug for marketing.

Additional insights into the Office of Biostatistics' most up-to-date thinking can be found in the statistical reviews and evaluations written by their statisticians during the review of NDAs. Once drugs are approved, these reports become public domain documents, allowing a window into the FDA statisticians' thinking.

2.8 THE COMMON TECHNICAL DOCUMENT

The common technical document (CTD) is a method of submitting an NDA. It is a very useful outcome of ICH discussions regarding the creation and implementation of standardized document formats. While individual regulatory agencies still have different requirements of specific content of various documents, this standardized format is a considerable step forward in the harmonization of submissions to multiple agencies. This guideline, adopted by the ICH regions (Europe, Japan, and the United States) in 2000, has subsequently been implemented, and other countries may continue to adopt it.

The CTD consists of five modules, although it must be noted that module 1 is technically not part of the CTD since it is region specific and may contain quite different information from one regulatory submission to another. Module 2 contains a brief general introduction and summary information addressing manufacturing issues (quality) and the safety and efficacy of the drug. Module 3 contains information on quality, and modules 4 and 5 contain individual study reports for nonclinical studies and clinical studies, respectively.

A further development related to the CTD is the move toward submitting it electronically, a submission format called e-CTD that was initiated through the ICH. In this format, information is contained in individual files that are associated with a “backbone.” In this way, information that is submitted as part of one application can be used in another application simply by providing information concerning where it is “located” in the sponsor’s accumulating database. The FDA actively encourages NDA submission in the e-CTD format. ICH Guideline M4, The CTD, provides more information on this submission format.

PART II

DRUG DISCOVERY AND NONCLINICAL RESEARCH

3

Drug Discovery

3.1 Introduction

Historically, many pharmaceutical agents were naturally occurring chemical substances, and discovery of their medicinally beneficial properties was serendipitous rather than deliberate. In the last several decades, research scientists have evaluated many molecules in a systematic manner and discovered drug molecules with interesting pharmacological characteristics. It was quite possible that hundreds (if not thousands) of potential drug candidate molecules would be made and tested for pharmacodynamic action in what was a very laborious process. Natural products and synthetic organic products, both of which are small molecules, were the typical drugs brought to market. The development of antihypertensive drugs and cholesterol lowering drugs fall neatly into this research and development (R&D) model. The plasma cholesterol lowering drug mevastatin is a drug derived from natural products. It is a fungal metabolite and one of the "statins" that lowers cholesterol by inhibiting the enzyme human growth hormone coenzyme A (HMG CoA) reductase (Rang, 2006a).

3.1.1 Small-Molecule Drug Candidates

More recently, as biomedical science has advanced rapidly and knowledge of molecular chemistry and molecular biology has increased dramatically, small-molecule drug discovery has become more technology driven. The starting point in recent small-molecule drug development is often knowledge of the molecular structure of the drug's biological target, the target receptor, which is typically a macromolecule (see Section 3.2.1). Given this knowledge, molecular technologies are utilized to discover a drug whose molecular structure is appropriate to facilitate the desired pharmacological effect. Additionally, the term "drug design" has become common. Drug design is concerned with modifying the structure of an existing chemical molecule in specific ways, including modification of its pharmacokinetic profile or synthesizing a related new chemical molecule specifically for its pharmacological benefit. (See also Fischer and Ganellin, 2006.)

While the concept of drug design has become a very attractive one, Mitscher and Dutta (2006) observed that desirable characteristics, such as an advantageous pharmacokinetic profile, can be difficult to engineer into a drug molecule at satisfactory levels. Therefore, while pursuing drug design, it is still very worthwhile to look for drug molecules that are likely to possess satisfactory pharmacokinetic profiles initially, i.e., molecules that are "intrinsically druglike" (Mitscher and Dutta, 2006).

New Drug Development: Design, Methodology, and Analysis. By J. Rick Turner

The ultimate goals of drug discovery and design are to identify a lead compound, a drug molecule that is the first-choice candidate for the next stage of the drug development process (nonclinical testing) and then to optimize the molecule. This latter activity is called lead optimization. It refers to searching for a closely related molecule or chemically engineering modifications in the lead drug molecule to identify the molecule that is best suited to progress to nonclinical testing.

3.1.2 Biopharmaceutical Drug Candidates

Biopharmaceuticals comprise another very important category of molecules that have beneficial therapeutic properties. Biopharmaceuticals will be considered separately for several reasons. First, the drug discovery process is different. Second, there are important differences in the pharmacokinetics and pharmacodynamic properties of traditional small-molecule drugs and biopharmaceuticals. While general pharmacokinetic and pharmacodynamic principles apply equally to small-molecule drugs and biopharmaceutical drugs, biopharmaceuticals often exhibit unique pharmacokinetic and pharmacodynamic properties (Meibohm, 2006). Discussion of biopharmaceuticals starts in Section 3.6.

3.2 OVERVIEW OF PHARMACEUTICS, PHARMACOKINETICS, AND PHARMACODYNAMICS

Before discussing drug discovery and design it is appropriate to introduce three topics: pharmaceutics, pharmacokinetics, and pharmacodynamics. In drug therapy there are three phases that need to be considered: the pharmaceutical phase, in which a drug molecule is administered to the body; the pharmacokinetic phase, during which the drug molecule travels around the body to the vicinity of its target receptor; and the pharmacodynamic phase, in which the drug molecule interacts with the target receptor. These are considered here in reverse order. Before doing this, however, we will address the concept of a receptor, since receptors feature prominently in future discussions.

3.2.1 Drug Receptors

Most drugs exert their influence by associating with specific macromolecules, often located in the surface membrane of a cell, in ways that alter the macromolecules' biochemical or biophysiological activities. This idea, which is more than a century old, is embodied in the term "receptor." A receptor is regarded as the component(s) of a cell or organism that interacts with a drug and initiates the chain of biochemical events leading to the drug's observed effects (Bourne and von Zastrow, 2004). The receptor concept has proved incredibly useful in molecular biology for explaining many aspects of biological regulation, and receptors have become a central focus of investigation in the areas of pharmacodynamics and the molecular basis of drug action.

As Bourne and von Zastrow (2004) noted, the receptor concept has important practical consequences for the development of new drugs:

- Receptors largely determine the quantitative relations between the concentration of a drug in the body and its pharmacological effects.
- Receptors are responsible for the selectivity of a drug's action. The molecular size, shape, and electrical charge of a drug determine whether, and with what affinity, it will bind to a particular receptor: There are an enormous amount of chemically different receptors. This means that the chemical structure of a new drug can dramatically increase or decrease its affinities for different classes of receptors, with resulting alterations in therapeutic and toxic effects.
- Receptors mediate the actions of both pharmacological agonists and antagonists. Agonists activate the receptor to produce a physiological signal as a direct result of binding to it. Antagonists bind to a receptor but do not activate a signal. However, this binding has a very important consequence: Other drugs that could have interacted with the receptor and caused a physiological signal are no longer able to. That is, antagonists interfere with the ability of an agonist to activate the cell. While the discussions in this book focus on developing a new drug that exerts a direct effect, i.e., the new drug is an agonist, it should be noted that pharmacological antagonists also play an important role in clinical medicine.

Most receptors are proteins. Wishart (2005) noted that proteins are perhaps the most complex chemical entities in nature: "No other class of molecule exhibits the variety and irregularity in shape, size, texture, and mobility than can be found in proteins" (proteins are discussed in more detail in Chapter 14). The tremendous diversity in proteins, and their specificity of shape and electrical charge, may be the reason for the evolution of their role as receptors. The best-characterized receptors are regulatory proteins. Regulatory proteins mediate the actions of endogenous messengers such as neurotransmitters and hormones, and this class of receptors mediates the effects of many of the most useful therapeutic agents (Bourne and von Zastrow, 2004).

3.2.2 The Pharmacodynamic Phase

Pharmacodynamics is the study of the effect that a drug has on the body, such as lowering blood pressure (Mitscher and Dutta, 2006). The pharmacodynamic phase begins once the drug molecule reaches the microenvironment of its target receptor. Once the drug molecule is in this region, it has the chance to approach the receptor, to dock with it, and to exert its pharmacological effect. A drug molecule has various functional units, as does a drug receptor. The ability of a drug molecule to dock with its target receptor is facilitated by the fact that the molecular geometries of the drug's functional groups and the receptor's functional groups are complementary. This docking, also known as binding, allows the electrons of the drug's functional groups to interact with the electrons of the receptor's functional groups, thus enabling an energetic interaction to occur and a pharmacological (biological) effect to be exerted.

3.2.3 The Pharmacokinetic Phase

In order for a drug molecule to have the opportunity to exert its pharmacodynamic effect, the drug molecule needs to reach its target receptor, which may be deep within the body. This means that a drug molecule must be able to travel within the body and traverse various physiological obstacles to successfully reach its target. Pharmacokinetics is the study of the effect that the body has on the drug. The pharmacokinetic phase can be defined as the time from the drug's absorption into the body until it reaches the microenvironment of the receptor site (Nogrady and Weaver, 2005).

Various characteristics of the molecule influence its chances of reaching its target receptor since they influence the nature and extent of the body's effect on it. A drug's pharmacokinetic profile therefore determines the extent of the drug's opportunity to exert its pharmacodynamic effect. While there are various routes for human drug administration (oral; rectal; intravenous, subcutaneous, intramuscular, and intra-arterial injections; topical; and direct inhalation into the lungs), the most common for small-molecule drugs is oral administration, and discussions in the first part of this chapter therefore focus on oral administration. (In contrast, biopharmaceuticals are typically administered by injection, often directly into the bloodstream.)

Dhillon and Gill (2006) defined pharmacokinetics as "a fundamental scientific discipline that underpins applied therapeutics" and noted that pharmacokinetics "provides a mathematical basis to assess the time course of drugs and their effects in the body." Four pharmacokinetic processes that determine the concentration of a drug that has been administered are:

- Absorption.
- Distribution.
- Metabolism.
- Elimination.

Research scientists involved in drug discovery/design and development are aware that understanding pharmacokinetic and concentration-response relationships is extremely beneficial, and knowledge from these areas is now being applied extensively in this area (Tozer and Rowland, 2006). The chemical structure of the drug can have a profound influence on how the drug performs its intended mission, i.e., achieving a biological effect by reaching its target receptor and interacting with it in a pharmacodynamic manner.

Metabolism is of particular interest here. Humans are exposed to a wide array of foreign compounds, or xenobiotics, every day. Many of these xenobiotics are ingested, while others enter via the lungs or the skin. Processed foods, for example, contain a large amount of xenobiotics. Fortunately, the body is very good at getting rid of these foreign substances, and it has sophisticated methods for neutralizing and eliminating them. However, these sophisticated neutralization and elimination methods are problematic in the case of drugs, which are also xenobiotics and are therefore subject to the same actions by the body.

Metabolism in the liver and excretion by the kidneys are two of the body's main neutralization and elimination strategies. Drug discovery/design has to take these methods into account, since a potentially effective drug, i.e., one with a good pharmacodynamic profile indicating successful interaction with its target receptor, will not be clinically useful if it does not actually reach the target receptor in the chemical state necessary to affect the desired therapeutic response.

3.2.4 The Pharmaceutical Phase

The pharmaceutical phase can be defined as the time from the point of administration of the drug molecule until it is absorbed into the circulation of the body (Nogrady and Weaver, 2005). As noted, discussions regarding small-molecule drugs involve oral administration of drugs. In this case, the pharmaceutical phase is the time from placing the drug in the mouth until it is absorbed across the intestinal wall into the gastrointestinal tract.

Drugs that are administered orally need to have certain properties in order to be a practical option for pharmacological therapy. The active pharmaceutical ingredient (API), the drug molecule that will eventually exert the drug's pharmacodynamic effects, is likely to be a very small component of the tablet. Various other nonpharmacologically active ingredients, called excipients, are also constituents of the tablet. Each of these excipients has a specific characteristic that enables it to perform a useful function in getting the API to its target receptor.

The pharmaceutical scientist needs to consider the drug product's formulation. A tablet is actually a complex, manufactured "drug molecule delivery system" that gets the drug molecule safely through the first part of its journey to its target receptor. Some of the excipients protect the drug molecule from various potential chemical attacks that will affect the molecule's chemical structure as it travels from the mouth to the gastrointestinal tract and into the body's fluids. Others help it to travel through the gastrointestinal tract without sticking and then to release the API so that it can be absorbed in the small intestine. At this point, the drug is said to be released from its formulation.

3.3 MEDICINAL CHEMISTRY

The interdisciplinary science of medicinal chemistry provides "a molecular bridge between the basic science of biology and the clinical science of medicine" (Norgrady and Weaver, 2005). It focuses on the discovery/design of new molecular entities, their optimization, and their development as useful drug molecules for the treatment of disease. These authors provide a comprehensive definition of a useful drug. A useful drug molecule has the following properties:

- It is safe.
- It is efficacious.
- It can successfully navigate all necessary regulatory oversight, including those that govern nonclinical trials and human clinical trials, and be approved by regulatory agencies for marketing.
- It can be manufactured in sufficiently large quantities by processes that can comply with all necessary regulatory oversight and that are financially viable for the sponsor.
- It can be successfully marketed and therefore be prescribed by clinicians.
- It can help individuals with a specified disease (and possibly other diseases too in the future).

This list of drug properties provides an excellent framework for the discussions in the following chapters.

3.3.1 Drug Molecules

A molecule is the essence of a substance. It is the smallest unit of that substance that still retains the substance's chemical identity. The atoms within a molecule can be conceptualized as being grouped into various molecular components called functional groups. A common functional group in acidic molecules is the carboxylic acid group, represented in the language of atoms as "–COOH." This functional group consists of a carbon atom, two oxygen atoms, and a hydrogen atom. Functional groups determine the chemical and physical properties of molecules.

Druglike molecules possess certain characteristics. For example, they have a relatively low molecular weight and possess one or more functional groups that are held together on a structural framework or "backbone." This backbone needs to be relatively rigid to ensure that the shape of the molecule does not alter too much. The functional groups are therefore positioned in three-dimensional space in a specific geometrical array and are available to interact with macromolecules. The term "druglike molecule" is used for a molecule that could theoretically be a match for a receptor site on a macromolecule. The term "drug molecule" is used once it is known that the molecule is a match for, i.e., it will bind with, a specific receptor site. A receptor that might be a useful target for a drug is called a druggable target until it is known to be useful, at which point it becomes a drug target.

3.3.2 Macromolecules, Receptors, and Drug Targets

Endogenous macromolecules are common in mammalian cells. Two examples are proteins and nucleic acids. An important characteristic of macromolecules is that they can be receptors and hence druggable targets and ultimately drug targets. Conceptually, receptors contain sites to which a functional unit on a drug molecule can attach; the three-dimensional shape of the functional unit is a match for the structure of the receptor site. The term "druggable target" is used for receptors that have sites which could theoretically be a match for a drug molecule. The term "drug target" is used once it is known that a specific drug molecule will attach to, i.e., bind with, the receptor site.

3.3.3 Structure-Activity Considerations and Drug-Receptor Interactions

Since the advent of computer-aided structure-activity modeling, the term "pharmacophore" has become a common and useful concept when describing drug-receptor interactions and when discussing the process of drug design. A pharmacophore is "the ensemble of steric and electronic features that is necessary to ensure the optimal supramolecular interactions with a specific biological target structure and to trigger (or to block) its biological response" [International Union of Pure and Applied Chemistry (IUPAC), cited by Wermuth, 2006].

A drug molecule can be regarded as a "collection of molecular fragments held in a three-dimensional arrangement that determines and defines all of the properties of the drug molecule" (Nogrady and Weaver, 2005). These properties include physiochemical, shape and stereochemical, and electronic properties, properties mentioned in the definition of a pharmacophore provided in the previous paragraph. These properties are important in determining whether a drug molecule that is administered to an individual will reach the drug target and will then interact with the drug target successfully. The influences of these properties can be outlined as follows (Nogrady and Weaver, 2005):

- Physiochemical. Physiochemical properties impact a drug's solubility and pharmacokinetic characteristics, influencing the drug's ability to reach the region of the body in which the drug target is located, which can be a long way from the site of the drug's administration. For example, the blood-brain barrier must be successfully crossed for a drug to bind to a receptor site in the brain.
- Shape and stereochemical. These properties affect the pharmacodynamic phase of drug action and influence the drug's interaction with its target receptor. Shape and stereochemical properties describe the structural arrangement of the drug molecule's constituent atoms and influence the molecule's final approach toward the target receptor.
- Electronic. Electronic properties also affect the pharmacodynamic phase of drug action. The electronic properties of a molecule are governed by the

distribution of electrons within the molecule. These properties determine the exact nature of the binding interaction that occurs between the drug and its target receptor and the degree to which the interaction is energetically favorable. The energetic exchange that occurs between the drug molecule and the receptor determines the strength of the biological signal that is generated. It is this signal that governs the physiological (pharmacological) effects of the drug.

An overview of these drug molecule properties allows further consideration of the definition of a pharmacophore provided two paragraphs previously (Wermuth, 2006):

- A pharmacophore does not represent an actual molecule or an actual association of functional groups. Rather, it is a purely abstract concept that accounts for the common molecular interaction capacities of a group of compounds toward their target structure.
- It describes the essential (steric and electronic) function-determining points necessary for an optimal interaction with a relevant target.
- It can be considered as the highest common denominator of a group of molecules exhibiting a similar pharmacological profile and which are recognized by the same target receptor.

In a similar manner, a toxicophore is conceptualized as an assembly of geometrical and electronic features of a different functional group of atoms in the drug molecule that interacts with a nontarget receptor and elicits an unwanted biological response, or side effect. Another relevant fragment of the drug is termed the "metabophore": This is the three-dimensional arrangement of atoms that is responsible for the molecule's metabolic properties. In this context, therefore, drug molecules are multiphores that consist of various biophores, biologically functional groups, located on a structural framework that is typically an organic molecule (Nogrady and Weaver, 2005).

Once the drug molecule enters the microenvironment of the target receptor, it is necessary that the geometry of the molecule precisely matches the geometry of the receptor site on the target receptor molecule. The pharmacophore therefore needs to be spatially and geometrically positioned consistently as the drug molecule approaches the target receptor.

In some molecules, the same set of atoms that comprise the molecule can be arranged in more than one way. The term "isomer" is used to describe each of the different versions of such a molecule. The term "conformational isomerism" is used to describe the process whereby a molecule undergoes transitions from one shape. The physical properties of the molecule remain the same; it is simply the shape that has changed. This means that some versions of the molecule will be optimally suited to interact with the receptor site, while other versions may be less optimally suited, and other versions not at all suited.

3.4 CHEMINFORMATICS, BIOINFORMATICS, AND COMPUTER-AIDED MOLECULAR DESIGN

Modern computing techniques are increasingly being used in drug discovery and design. Two recent trends have facilitated this paradigm shift. First, the phenomenal growth in information from molecular biological studies provides the pharmaceutical industry with tremendous opportunities to capitalize on this information in the development of new drugs. This includes a knowledge of how genetic material codes for the production of proteins, knowledge of the structure and function of proteins, how proteins create metabolic pathways, and how environmental factors affect the phenotypic expression of a person's genotype to create a unique individual human being with a unique set of metabolic pathways.

The second trend is a tremendous advancement in computing systems (often sophisticated networks of relatively small computers rather than hugely powerful individual machines). The combination of advances in these areas has facilitated the development of cheminformatics and bioinformatics, highly computational fields that deal with storing and communicating the ever-increasing amount of molecular chemical and molecular biological data available. While bioinformatics employs tremendous computing power, it is important to emphasize that it is, at heart, a biological discipline.

3.4.1 Bioinformatics

Bioinformatics is at the heart of understanding the workings of the cell. The vast amounts of information from many subdisciplines within molecular and cell biology need to be integrated into a cellular model that can be used to generate hypotheses for testing (Bader and Enright, 2005). As these authors commented:

> Bioinformatics will play a vital role in overcoming this data integration and modeling challenge, because databases, visualization software, and analysis software must be built to enable data assimilation and to make the results accessible and useful for answering biological questions (p. 254).

Historically, *in vitro* and *in vivo* testing has been the mainstay of evaluating a drug molecule's action and testing various iterations in the process of the molecule's optimization. The advent of tremendously powerful computers and computer clusters has changed many aspects of drug discovery and development and has facilitated another approach known as *in silico* testing. Before a molecule is even synthesized, extensive computer modeling takes place in an attempt to identify a molecule that has a high probability of achieving the desired interaction with a target receptor. *In silico* development focuses on many aspects of the molecule, including its ability to reach the region of the drug receptor, its ability to approach and dock (bind) with the receptor, and particularly the precise nature of the binding interaction with the target receptor. It is also concerned with binding interactions with nontarget receptors, which lead to adverse events.

Knowledge of the structure of the receptor macromolecule now permits research scientists to adapt the approaches of computer-assisted design to create the field of computer-assisted molecular design (CAMD). In combination with the disciplines of bioinformatics and cheminformatics, it has become possible to design lead compounds from scratch that are probabilistically well suited for further development and optimization. CAMD facilitates *in silico* three-dimensional docking experiments, i.e., simulations of potential drug molecules docking with receptors. The results of these experiments can identify a potentially safe and efficacious drug molecule relatively more easily, cheaply, and quickly than other approaches in drug discovery.

As a lead compound is optimized, enhancing the features of the pharmacophore in order to elicit a more energetic therapeutic interaction with the receptor is important. So too is modifying toxicophores to lessen or eliminate side effects. In addition to these pharmacodynamic and toxicodynamic considerations, pharmacokinetic considerations need to be addressed. The goal here is to modify the metabophore where possible to minimize the drug's metabolism in the liver and its rapid excretion by the kidneys, thereby giving the molecule a greater chance to exert its desired pharmacodynamic effects.

In addition to exploring the nature and properties of useful drug molecules, investigating the structure and function of the other half of the pharmacodynamic equation, the receptor macromolecule, is important. Knowledge of the structure of the receptor macromolecule now permits research scientists to design lead compounds from scratch that are probabilistically well suited for further development and optimization.

3.5 FUTURE TRENDS IN SMALL-MOLECULE DRUG DEVELOPMENT

Despite increased R&D expenditure and pharmaceutical companies' historical familiarity with the developmental process of small-molecule drugs, the flow of new small-molecule drugs seems to be decreasing (Rang and LeVine, 2006). Two fundamental problems are as follows. First, the inherent "foreign nature" of chemically synthesized compounds presents a problem once the drug is administered: As noted earlier, humans have very good mechanisms for eliminating xenobiotics. Second, prediction of a drug's toxicity profile once the drug is marketed and taken by a large number of patients is extremely difficult. Even large-scale clinical trials do not forecast the occurrence and prevalence of relatively rare side effects that can be seen once the drug is widely available (see Chapter 13). This issue can lead to withdrawal of drugs from the market, either voluntarily or after regulatory intervention.

Nevertheless, small-molecule drugs will likely continue to play a major role in medical treatment (Rang and LeVine, 2006). First, many small-molecule drugs have been very successful therapeutically. Second, major pharmaceutical companies have large libraries of small-molecule compounds that have druglike properties. With the advantages of new technologies such as combinatorial chemistry (see Ross, McNaughton, and Miller, 2005), high-throughput screening (see Banks et al., 2005; Homon and Nelson, 2006), and genomic approaches to target identification (see Primrose and Twyman, 2004), these libraries will help companies continue to develop small-molecule drugs.

3.6 BIOPHARMACEUTICALS

Biopharmaceuticals are large-molecule drugs, or macromolecule drugs. The term "biopharmaceutical" was originally coined to define "therapeutic proteins produced by genetic engineering, rather than by extraction from normal biological sources" (LeVine, 2006). The importance of genetic engineering in this context is the production of large quantities of particular proteins that are otherwise difficult to obtain. This includes proteins that are present only in human cells (Hartl and Jones, 2006).

Walsh (2003) defined biopharmaceuticals as therapeutic protein or nucleic acid preparations made by techniques involving recombinant deoxyribonucleic acid (DNA) technology. Therapeutic proteins include blood clotting factors and plasminogen activators, hemopoietic factors, hormones, interferons and interleukins, and monoclonal antibodies (LeVine, 2006). Over time, the term "biopharmaceutical" has broadened, and, in addition to proteins and nucleic acids, now includes bacteriophages, viral and bacterial vaccines, vectors for gene therapy, and cells for cell therapy (Primrose and Twyman, 2004). Attention here focuses on proteins, since the majority of approved biopharmaceuticals are proteins.

3.6.1 Molecular Genetics and Proteins

In higher organisms, including human beings, biological information flows in a particular manner. Instructions coded in the genetic material DNA undergo transcription and translation by ribonucleic acid (RNA) and are then delivered to the protein assembly machinery. While the acronym DNA has become embedded in modern language, the acronym RNA has received less attention. This discrepancy is arguably unfortunate, as RNA too is critical to life as we know it.

As Bryson (2003) commented, "It is a notable oddity of biology that DNA and proteins don't speak the same language." Watson (2004) addressed this issue more formally. For some time following the identification of the molecular structure of DNA (see Watson and Crick, 1953), there was puzzlement concerning this apparent contradiction:

> The prevailing assumption that the original life-form consisted of a DNA molecule posed an inescapable contradiction: DNA

> cannot assemble itself; it requires proteins to do so. Which came first? Proteins, which have no known means of duplicating information, or DNA, which can duplicate information but only in the presence of proteins? The problem was insoluble: you cannot, we thought, have DNA without proteins, and you cannot have proteins without DNA (p. 84).

An answer to this apparent riddle is provided by RNA. Ribonucleic acid is actually a DNA equivalent, since it can store and replicate genetic information. Importantly, it is also a protein equivalent, since it can catalyze critical chemical reactions. Indeed, the first life-forms were probably entirely RNA based, and RNA has remained part of our cellular systems (Watson, 2004). Thus, RNA translates the genetic information coded for in our DNA into information that proteins can understand and act upon and does so in a remarkable manner.

In the mid-1970s, it was generally accepted that genes existed as continuous segments within a DNA molecule. This view changed radically with the discovery in 1977 that, in higher organisms (eukaryotic cells), an individual gene can comprise several DNA segments separated by chunks of noncoding DNA (see Roberts, 1993). An elegant editing process called RNA splicing removes these noncoding chunks of genetic material and connects the relevant segments together to create messenger RNA. Messenger RNA then ensures that amino acids are successfully made. Amino acids are joined together in various sequences to make proteins. Proteins are therefore made from the genetic instructions coded in the DNA molecule.

Proteins have many biological functions. Of particular relevance in this book are their function as drug receptors and their function as enzymes. Enzymes are the largest class of proteins. Virtually all enzyme names end in "-ase." Enzymes act as catalysts for almost all of the chemical reactions that occur in living organisms. Almost all steps in biological reactions, therefore, are catalyzed by enzymes. It is thought that enzymes reduce the activation energy required for each of the stages in these reactions by a considerable amount (Thomas, 2003).

3.6.2 Protein Structures

A protein is actually much more than the linear chain of amino acid residues that comprise it. As Wishart (2005) commented, proteins are perhaps the most complex chemical entities in nature: "No other class of molecule exhibits the variety and irregularity in shape, size, texture, and mobility than can be found in proteins." This degree of complexity is captured in a hierarchical model that best represents current efforts to simplify their description and look for structural commonalities. There are various levels in this hierarchical model.

The primary structure represents the sequence of a protein, the string of amino acids that comprise it. The individual amino acids in this chain are termed "residues," and these residues are joined together (covalently connected together) by peptide bonds to form chains. This string of amino acids is shapeless and not biologically active. The nature of the chemical bonds and the chemical nature of various amino acid side chains mean that proteins do not exist simply as an extended string of amino acids. As Wishart (2005) expressed it, "proteins have a natural proclivity to form more complex structures."

Secondary structures are formed by short stretches of residues. These substructures make up sequentially proximal components of proteins, and they have shapes. There are various forms of protein secondary structures, e.g., helices (the most common of which is the α-helix), β-sheets, β-turns, Ω–loops, and some that remain unclassifiable and are typically referred to as random coil or loop regions. A complex combination of attractive and repulsive forces between close and more distant parts of the structure affects the resultant shape of secondary structures, and predicting secondary structure from knowledge of the linear amino acid sequence alone remains a tremendous challenge.

The overall three-dimensional structure of a protein is called the tertiary structure. The tertiary structure represents the "spatial packing" of secondary structures (Ofran and Rost, 2005). As for secondary structures, there are several different classes of tertiary structures. More advanced classification schemes take into account "common topologies, motifs, or folds" (Wishart, 2005). Common tertiary folds include the α/β–barrel, the four-helix bundle, and the Greek key (we will discuss protein folding further in Chapter 14). Any change to any part of the structure of a protein will have an impact on its biological activity (Thomas, 2003).

3.6.3 Recombinant DNA Technology

DNA molecules are very large, and this size caused considerable problems in the early days of molecular biology. Understanding the precise function of particular stretches of DNA required isolating that part of the DNA molecule and then obtaining enough of it to work with. As Watson (2004) commented:

> In essence we needed a molecular editing system: a pair of molecular scissors that could cut the DNA text into manageable sections; a kind of molecular glue pot that would allow us to manipulate those pieces; and finally a molecular duplicating machine to amplify the pieces that we had cut out and isolated (pp. 87-88).

In 1973 many earlier discoveries came together in the form of recombinant DNA technology, "the capacity to edit DNA" (Watson, 2004).

Enzymes can be used to create fragments of DNA, and to join different fragments together. Restriction enzymes can cut DNA molecules internally at defined positions, creating predictable fragments with specific DNA sequences. Other enzymes called DNA ligases can join DNA fragments together. The novel arrangements created in this manner are called recombinant DNA molecules. To study these experimentally in a laboratory requires many copies. Recombinant

DNA technology facilitated the preparation of millions of copies of a given DNA sequence via the technique of molecular cloning (Primrose and Twyman, 2004).

3.6.4 Recombinant Proteins as Drugs

Among the first commercial biopharmaceutical applications of recombinant DNA technology was the synthesis of the proteins human growth hormone and insulin. There was a large demand for these, but "in many cases the authentic product had to be isolated from human cadavers or animals and there was a risk of contamination with pathogens" (Primrose and Twyman, 2004). The first recombinant proteins were produced in bacteria, which worked well for these simple proteins, and bacterial fermentation is still used in biopharmaceutical manufacture (see Chapter 12). More complex recombinant human proteins are produced in various ways, including large scale mammalian cell cultures. Recombinant subunit vaccines, such as hepatitis B and influenza vaccines, can be produced in yeast. The organisms that carry the recombinant genes and in which recombinant DNA drugs are produced are called host organisms.

3.6.5 Discovery and Development of Biopharmaceuticals

Most biopharmaceuticals have been discovered as a direct consequence of increased knowledge and understanding of the body's molecular mechanisms: Continuing advances in the molecular sciences "have deepened our understanding of the molecular mechanisms which underlie health and disease" (Walsh, 2003). While nature has optimized protein structures for their natural biological activities, these natural structures may not be optimal for pharmaceutical applications. Protein drug discovery typically starts with known biomolecules and the intent to modify them in certain ways to achieve certain desirable characteristics and activities. Genetic engineering is therefore employed to re-engineer the protein structure to enhance pharmaceutical characteristics (LeVine, 2006).

The discovery process for biopharmaceuticals, typically human proteins, is typically shorter and easier than it is for the small-molecule drugs discussed in earlier sections in this chapter. It is closely allied to the logical application of our rapidly expanding knowledge of the body's molecular functions. Screening and lead optimization are not required. In addition, the risks of immune responses to foreign molecules are essentially removed. The tremendous advances in genomics (the systematic study of the entire genome) and particularly proteomics (the study of all of a genome's putative proteins: see Chapter 14) will likely enhance this discovery process too, likely resulting in the identification of previously unidentified proteins that are potential biopharmaceuticals (Walsh, 2003).

The development of biopharmaceuticals shares some of the challenges of small-molecule drugs and also has some additional challenges. A challenge shared with small-molecule drugs is that *in vitro* tests and *in vivo* animal studies may not accurately predict the physiological response seen in humans with the disease or condition of interest. Additional challenges include finding effective ways of getting the drug to the appropriate location in the body. They may also have short plasma half-lives. Almost all biopharmaceuticals currently approved are given via injection (parenteral administration). This can be an issue in patient adherence (sticking to the prescribed treatment regimen). Having an injection infrequently is not particularly problematic, but frequent administration can be painful, inconvenient, and a cause of relatively poor adherence. Alternative routes of administration (e.g., oral, nasal, pulmonary) have not worked at all well so far for protein biopharmaceuticals. The high enzyme concentration in the gastrointestinal tract leads to inactivation, and their large size (high molecular mass) leads to low permeability through the gastrointestinal mucosa.

The interpretation and assessment of the pharmacokinetics of protein biopharmaceuticals often pose additional challenges compared to small-molecule drug candidates, therefore requiring additional resources. In general, these biopharmaceutical drug candidates are subject to the same general principles of pharmacokinetics, but their similarity to endogenous molecules can cause considerable complications in the evaluation of pharmacokinetics and pharmacokinetic/pharmacodynamic relationships (Meibohm, 2006).

3.7 CLINICAL TRIALS FOR SMALL-MOLECULE AND BIOPHARMACEUTICAL DRUG CANDIDATES

This chapter has provided an overview of some of the advances in drug discovery of both small-molecule and biopharmaceutical drugs. The increased knowledge we have concerning molecular chemistry, molecular biology, and the molecular basis of health and disease can confer considerable advantages in the drug discovery process. However, even with all of these sophisticated strategies working in the research scientist's favor, a drug candidate's pharmacokinetic and pharmacodynamic activity in humans cannot be precisely specified by *in silico*, *in vitro*, and animal testing. This means that the clinical trial methodology that is the focus of this book is still absolutely essential to evaluate a new drug candidate's biological activity in humans and hence its safety and efficacy.

In the context of this book, it is particularly noteworthy that the design, methodology, and analysis components of clinical trials for small-molecule investigational drugs are the same as those for biopharmaceutical investigational drugs. In both cases, the same study designs, experimental methodology, and statistical analyses are employed, and the same rigorous approach is needed to provide optimum quality data with which to provide optimum quality answers to the research questions of interest.

4

Nonclinical Research

4.1 Introduction

This chapter provides an overview of the typical nonclinical studies conducted in a drug development program. Many of these studies are conducted under regulatory governance, and reports of them are included in regulatory submissions. Three areas of study are considered here: pharmacokinetics, pharmacology, and toxicology. The scientific rationale of the studies is addressed, along with appropriate regulatory guidance.

4.1.1 Reduction, Refinement, and Replacement of Laboratory Animal Studies

The use of animals in laboratory studies is an emotional topic for many people (and as an animal lover, this author can certainly empathize). However, the importance of information gained from animal studies in the development of medicines for humans cannot be overstated. The development programs for all modern medicines included nonclinical research, and this will also be critical in the future development of medicines that address the most serious human diseases. Currently, regulatory agencies require animal studies to be conducted, a requirement solely intended for the protection of human subjects in clinical trials and human patients in the future. Fortunately, research organizations around the world are aware of the balance of having to use animals in research and wanting to cure human disease. A set of standards known as the "3Rs" guides research scientists: These address the reduction, refinement, and replacement of laboratory animal studies.

The fundamental principle here is that animals are only used when there is no alternative. Researchers have an ethical duty (and in some countries, a legal one) to check all of the available scientific literature to determine if there is an alternative way of acquiring the information that would be gained from an animal study. Innovation in any field of investigation that allows information to be gained from alternative research methodology not involving animals is welcomed by the pharmaceutical industry.

4.2 Pharmacokinetics

The discipline of pharmacokinetics was introduced in Chapter 3 to facilitate discussions in the arena of drug discovery and design. It is addressed here in the context of nonclinical studies, and it will also be discussed in the clinical context in

New Drug Development: Design, Methodology, and Analysis. By J. Rick Turner

Chapter 10. This involvement of pharmacokinetic discussion throughout the book attests to its central importance in new drug development.

Nonclinical pharmacokinetic investigation is helpful when interpreting the data from safety (pharmacological) studies, and it also provides support for toxicology studies. While nonhuman pharmacokinetic parameters are not perfectly predictive of human pharmacokinetics, they do constitute meaningful quantitative data that improve the chances of selecting the correct range of safe doses to test in humans. This dose selection is critically important to the success of clinical trials.

4.2.1 Absorption

Absorption addresses the transfer of the drug compound from the site of administration into the bloodstream. Studies here are typically single-dose studies (repeat-dose studies will be done, but they often fall under the heading of Toxicology studies, discussed in Section 4.4). The same animal species is used in these studies as is used in pharmacological and toxicological studies, and the route of drug administration is typically the route intended for use in clinical studies.

The plasma concentration-time profile is informative here: This is shown in Figure 4.1. The shape of this profile differs according to whether or not the reaction proceeds at a rate governed by the concentration of the drug in the body (blood plasma). In zero-order reactions, the reaction proceeds at a constant rate not governed by the concentration of the drug in the plasma. In first-order reactions, the reaction proceeds at a rate that is governed by the concentration of the drug in the plasma. First-order reactions are typical for most therapeutic drugs used in clinical practice. Accordingly, Figure 4.1 shows a plasma concentration-time profile for a first-order reaction.

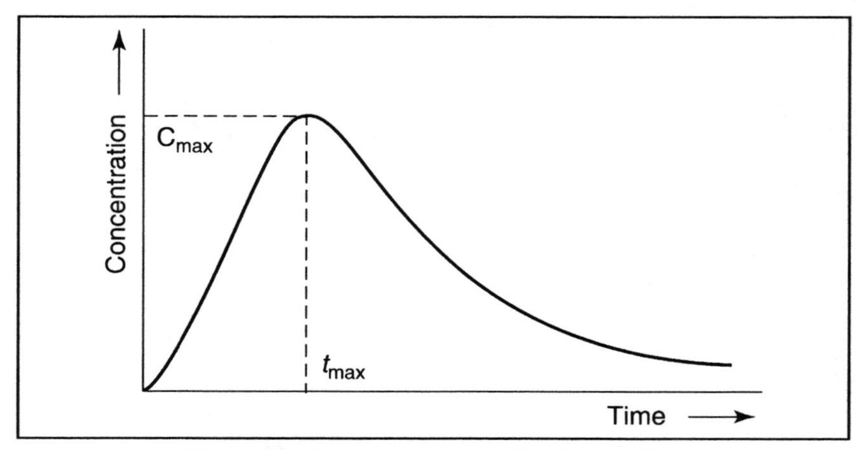

Figure 4.1. The plasma concentration-time profile.

Several quantitative pharmacokinetic terms are used to describe and quantify aspects of the plasma concentration-time profile of an administered drug (or its metabolites, which may or may not be pharmacologically active themselves). These include:

- C_{max}: The maximum concentration or maximum systemic exposure.
- T_{max}: The time of maximum concentration or time of maximum exposure.
- $t_{½}$, Half-life: The time required to reduce the plasma concentration to one-half of its initial value.
- AUC, Area under the plasma concentration curve over all time: A measure of total systemic exposure. $AUC_{(0\text{–}t)}$ denotes the area under the curve from zero to any time point t.

4.2.2 Distribution

ICH Guideline S3B addresses the typical format of distribution studies. The title of this guidance reflects that, while single-dose distribution studies are often sufficient, there are occasions when repeated-dose studies are warranted. This document states:

> A comprehensive knowledge of the absorption, distribution, metabolism, and elimination of a compound is important for the interpretation of pharmacology and toxicology studies. Tissue distribution studies are essential in providing information on distribution and accumulation of the compound and/or metabolites, especially in relation to potential sites of action; this information may be useful for designing toxicology and pharmacology studies and for interpreting the results of these experiments.

Distribution addresses the transfer of the drug compound from the site of administration to the systemic circulation and then to bodily tissues. Both *in vitro* and *in vivo* studies are informative here. *In vitro* studies, for example, examine plasma protein binding. *In vivo* studies use whole body autoradiography that can display visually how much drug has reached different parts of the body. Transfer of the drug compound in milk to an infant and across the placenta is also studied.

4.2.3 Metabolism

Metabolism addresses the biochemical transformation of a drug with the basic intent of eliminating it from the body: see Section 3.2.3.

4.2.4 Elimination

Excretion concerns the removal of the drug compound from the body. Both the original (parent) drug compound and its metabolites can be excreted. The primary mode of investigation here is excretion balance studies. Radiolabeled drug compound is administered and radioactivity is then measured from excretion sites (e.g., urine, feces, expired air). These studies provide information on which organs are involved in excretion and the time course of excretion.

4.3 PHARMACOLOGY

Pharmacology is the scientific discipline that specializes in the mechanisms of action, uses, and undesired effects of drugs. Pharmacology studies fall into two categories:

- Research pharmacology studies. These address primary and secondary pharmacology. They do not need to be performed to cGLP standards.
- Safety pharmacology studies. These studies examine physiological functional changes related to the drug compound's activity. They are performed to cGLP standards.

Each of these categories is considered in turn.

4.3.1 Research Pharmacology Studies

Research pharmacology studies are conducted at the start of a drug development program, and they fall outside the scope of regulatory governance. As noted above, they do not need to be performed to cGLP standards. The three regions of ICH classify the pharmacological actions of a drug into primary and secondary. Primary actions are related to the proposed therapeutic use, while secondary actions are not related.

Primary research pharmacology studies.

Primary pharmacology studies focus on the mechanism of action of the drug compound and can be conducted *in vitro* and/or *in vivo*. Studies conducted *in vitro* can include radioligand binding studies and focus on the drug's action at specific receptor sites in tissue preparations or in genetically engineered cell lines. Studies conducted *in vivo* investigate the potential pharmacological action of the drug in animal models as it relates to its intended therapeutic use.

The goal of primary pharmacology studies is to demonstrate that the drug compound has pharmacological (biological) activity relating to its proposed therapeutic use. Understanding a drug's mechanism of action is beneficial in several ways. It is useful in predicting potential safety issues and also in predicting potential interactions with other drugs that may be taken concomitantly by patients in the future. It can also provide clues to understanding undesired effects and in explaining the results of toxicology studies.

Secondary research pharmacology studies.

Secondary pharmacology studies focus on the overall pharmacological activity of the drug compound, activity that may occur that is not directly related to the drug's proposed therapeutic use. These studies can also be conducted *in vitro* and/or *in vivo*. Studies conducted *in vitro* include the drug molecule's likely binding with non-target receptors. Studies conducted *in vivo* investigate the general pharmacological action of the drug in animal models.

In addition to its intended therapeutic use, a drug may have other effects that can fall in several categories. Some of these may actually be beneficial, while others cause undesirable effects.

4.3.2 Safety Pharmacology Studies

As the name implies, safety pharmacology studies investigate potentially undesirable effects of the drug compound. While they are typically conducted in the rat and the dog, primate models can also be used. Typically, studies are single-dose studies using the intended therapeutic dose. These studies focus on functional changes in major organ systems within the body. Toxicology studies, addressed in Section 4.4, focus on structural changes. Issues of function and structure can be meaningfully separated here, although they can also be connected. Functional changes can occur in the absence of structural change, they can precede structural change, and they can potentially contribute to structural change.

Safety pharmacology studies investigate potentially undesirable effects of the drug compound on the physiological function of the central nervous system, the respiratory system, and the cardiovascular system. Some of the topics investigated are:

- Central nervous system: Skeletal muscle tone, locomotion, reflexes.
- Respiratory system: Rate and depth of breathing.
- Cardiovascular system: Blood pressure, heart rate, and electrophysiology, including electrocardiographic studies. Electrophysiological studies are conducted to examine the potential for QT interval prolongation.

4.3.3 QT Interval Prolongation

The QT interval can be seen on an electrocardiogram (ECG), as represented in Figure 4.2. The ECG is possibly the most recognized bodily pattern of activity. In the late nineteenth century, it was realized that the electrical changes occuring during the heart's contraction could be detected by placing electrodes on the skin and connecting them to a galvanometer. Early recording practices evolved via the pen-and-ink chart recorder to monitors that display the signals and to computerized systems that not only display the signals but concurrently digitize them and store them for later examination (Turner, 1994).

The ECG consists of the P-wave, the QRS complex, and the T-wave. These components, represented in Figure 4.2, are associated with different aspects of the cardiac cycle: atrial activity, excitation of the ventricles, and repolarization of the ventricles, respectively.

The actual length of the QT interval is a representation of its time, or duration, measured in milliseconds. A typical duration is in the order of 400–450 msec. However, in normal circumstances, as the heart beats faster (heart rate increases), the duration of an individual cardiac cycle decreases, since more cardiac cycles now occur in the same time. Therefore, as the cardiac cycle shortens, so do each of the components of the cardiac cycle. This means that the QT interval will naturally be shorter at a higher heart rate. Since it is of interest to examine the QT interval at various heart rates, the interval is "corrected" for heart rate, i.e., a term called QTc is calculated, by one of several methods.

QT interval prolongation can be congenital, and it can also be acquired, e.g., induced by drug therapy. QT interval prolongation (delayed ventricular repolarization) results in an increased risk of ventricular tachycardia, including a particular variant called torsade de pointes. Torsade de pointes is a life-threatening arrhythmia if a normal rhythm is not quickly restored, regardless of a person's prior cardiovascular history. Several drugs have been associated with QT prolongation and have caused drug-induced torsade de pointes, leading to their market withdrawal. Some drugs can cause QT prolongation within a normal dosing range.

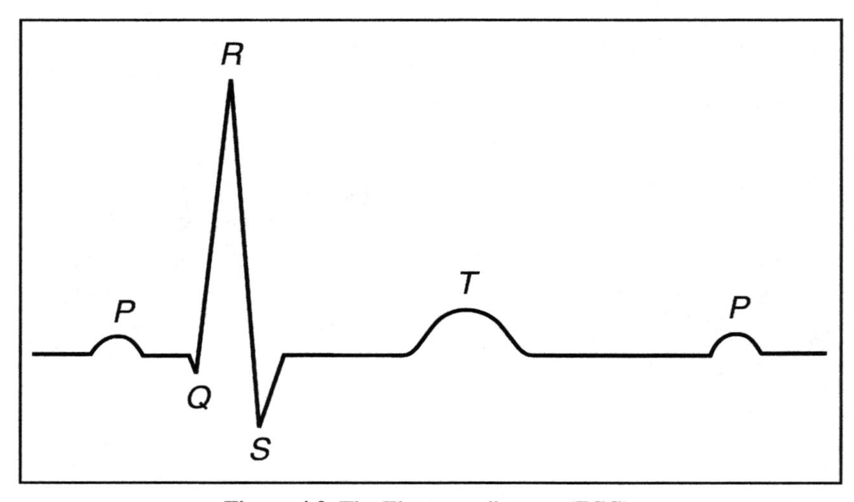

Figure 4.2. The Electrocardiogram (ECG).

In contrast, for other drugs, QT prolongation is only observed in the context of drug-drug interactions where the interaction causes an increase in the drug's serum concentration above the expected therapeutic range. For this reason, rigorous studies evaluating the influence of an investigational drug on ECG parameters as well as drug interaction studies are performed during nonclinical and clinical testing.

The case of Seldane provides an instructive illustration of a point made in Section 1.11. A drug needs to be reasonably safe, where "reasonably safe" can be thought of as representing an acceptable benefit/risk ratio. Identification of additional risk reduces this ratio (the denominator becomes larger). However, the benefit/risk ratio can also be reduced, i.e., made less acceptable, by decreasing the benefit (decreasing the numerator). The availability of other suitable drugs meant Seldane no longer offered a unique therapeutic benefit, and so the benefit component of the benefit/risk ratio decreased. This again worsened the benefit/risk ratio. As will be discussed in Chapter 13, many evaluations and decisions are necessary in drug therapy, and these are often not as simple as we might wish.

4.4 TOXICOLOGICAL STUDIES

As Gad (2006) commented, toxicology, like all other sciences, started as a descriptive science. Nonhuman animals and humans were dosed with various chemical agents and the resulting adverse effects observed and described. As the science matured, toxicology has also addressed mechanisms of action, and current studies often combine descriptive and mechanistic approaches. The use of statistics has also increased in this field. This section overviews nonclinical toxicological assessments and notes some similarities and differences in the statistical approaches employed here and those that are employed in clinical studies.

It is understood that the statistical approaches employed in clinical studies have not yet been discussed in detail, and therefore a more comprehensive understanding of the similarities and differences discussed here may be gained by rereading this section after reading Chapter 5 through Chapter 11. However, I have endeavored to make the discussions presented here as meaningful as possible at this point in the book.

4.4.1 Toxicodynamics

Drugs are categorized into classes. Different drugs belonging to the same class often have some toxicological effects in common, i.e., side effects that can be reasonably expected from all drugs in that class. However, it is also likely that each drug will have a unique toxicology profile, largely influenced by the drug's physiochemical properties (Hellman, 2006).

Most compounds that exert toxicological influences (toxicants) induce their effects by interacting with normal cellular processes (Hellman, 2006). The ultimate result of many toxic responses is cell death leading to loss of important organ function. Other toxicological effects are the result of interactions with various biochemical and physiological processes that do not affect the survival of the cells. Common mechanisms of toxic action include:

- Interference with cellular membrane functions.
- Disturbed calcium homeostasis.
- Disrupted cellular energy production.
- Reversible or nonreversible binding to various proteins, nucleic acids, and other macromolecules.

ICH Guidance M3(R1) addresses several topics related to toxicity, including single- and repeat-dose toxicity studies, genotoxicity, carcinogenicity, and reproductive toxicity. Relatively less evidence of toxicity is considered to imply relatively greater safety of the drug. The route of administration of the drug compound is the same as that intended in clinical settings (although, where particularly informative, other routes may be used to gain information that will be beneficial for clinical investigations).

The main phases of nonclinical toxicology assessment for a new synthetic drug, in chronological order, are as follows (Rang, 2006b):

- Exploratory toxicology studies.
- Regulatory toxicology studies performed before drug is administered to humans for the first time in FTIH studies.
- Regulatory toxicology studies performed in parallel with clinical trials.

4.4.2 Exploratory Toxicology Studies

The purpose of exploratory toxicology studies is to provide an idea of the main organs and physiological systems involved and a quantitative estimation of the drug's toxicity when administered, in single or repeated doses, across a relatively short period of time. These studies are typically not required to be reported to the regulatory agency prior to FTIH studies, do not need to be conducted according to cGLP guidelines, and are not typically conducted with a drug compound that has been manufactured to cGMP standards.

4.4.3 Pre-FTIH Regulatory Toxicology Studies

Full reports of all regulatory toxicology studies are submitted to the FDA and are accordingly conducted according to cGLP standards. Pre-FTIH regulatory toxicology studies are required before the drug is administered to humans for the first time. These include:

- Twenty-eight-day repeated-dose toxicology studies in two nonhuman animal species.
- Genotoxicity studies.
- Reproductive toxicity studies.
- Safety pharmacology studies.

4.4.4 Post-FTIH Regulatory Toxicology Studies

Other regulatory toxicology studies are typically conducted in parallel with clinical trials. These include:

- Toxicological studies in two or more nonhuman animal species lasting up to one year.
- Carcinogenicity tests and reproductive toxicology studies lasting up to two years.
- Interaction studies that examine possible drug-drug interactions with other drugs that may be prescribed concurrently in humans for the same indication for which the new drug is being developed.

Results from these studies are not the primary determinant of whether or not the drug progresses into FTIH studies, but once the drug has done so and may therefore reach the NDA stage, these data are required. The rationale for waiting to start these studies until the drug has a chance of marketing approval is largely financial. These studies are expensive to conduct, and, if the drug is not going to progress into FTIH studies, they are typically not done.

4.4.5 Dose Range-Finding Toxicology

The first of several stages of toxicological investigation involves a dose range-finding study conducted to estimate the "no toxic effect level," or NTEL. There are several possible designs. One comprises the administration (if possible, via the intended route of administration for humans) of a single dose at one particular dose level to each test animal. Several widely spaced doses are chosen, and the animals are observed daily for two weeks. Weight, morbidity, and visible signs of toxicity are noted, and animals that die during this period are autopsied. At the end of the two-week period, animals are sacrificed and autopsied to look for evidence of gross organ damage. Another design involves dose escalation, in which animals receive increasing doses until toxicity appears or a predetermined maximum dose is reached.

4.4.6 Genotoxicity

Mutation is a common and naturally occurring event, and most mutations do not lead to deleterious end results since nature has also produced very effective DNA repair mechanisms. Mutagenicity is the chemical alteration of DNA that is sufficient to cause abnormal gene expression. Mutagenicity, also known as genotoxicity, is a more comprehensive set of events, of which carcinogenicity and teratogenicity are very important subsets. Carcinogenicity describes activity that leads to cancer, and teratogenicity describes activity that leads to the impairment of fetal development. All new drug development now requires specified tests for reproductive and developmental toxicology, including teratogenicity. These tests include investigation of reproductive impairment, teratogenicity, and neurotoxicity at some time in the future following exposure to the test material.

Full nonclinical evaluation of carcinogenicity and teratogenicity require long-term animal studies. Given the expense of these, earlier *in vitro* testing for general signs of mutagenicity can be conduced in various ways, including the use of bacteria (the Ames test is a test of mutagenicity in *Salmonella typhimurium*) and mammalian cells. Newer tests provide a quicker and less expensive way of predicting whether a material is a mutagen, and possibly a carcinogen, than do longer *in vivo* animal tests, but they are not as conclusive (Gad, 2006).

4.5 DESIGN, METHODOLOGY, AND ANALYSIS CONSIDERATIONS

Nonclinical research provides very useful information and plays a considerable role in the successful development of a new drug. It is also required by current regulatory statutes. Nonetheless, no matter how meticulously, rigorously, and comprehensively nonclinical testing is conducted, no animal model is a perfect model of the drug's actions and effects in humans. Therefore, in addition to an appreciation of the usefulness of nonclinical data, it is valuable to have an appreciation of their limitations and of statistical considerations of particular pertinence to toxicological data.

Gad (2006) discussed several characteristics of toxicological data, including:

- Data are typically generated from relatively small sample sizes (there are ethical requirements to minimize sample sizes). Hence, the toxicologist deals with relatively small data sets that are not collected from the population of ultimate interest (humans).
- Investigation often involves dealing with data from a sample that was not able to provide all of the data that was intended by the study design. This can be the result of difficulties dealing with equipment handling, for example, cultured cells and bacterial cultures, and with test animal deaths.
- Experimental designs are not standardized, in that there is a tremendous range of possible studies, since the dose of drug chosen, the route of drug administration, the subject population, and the length of the study can all vary considerably.

These observations underline the fact that assessments of data from nonclinical toxicological experimentation "should be undertaken with full knowledge of the involved uncertainties, weaknesses, and difficulties" (Gad, 2006).

4.5.1 Randomization in Nonclinical Studies

The topic of randomization in clinical trials is addressed in the following chapter (see Section 5.6). Briefly, the randomization process involves randomly assigning subjects to one or other of the treatment groups to make the treatment groups as similar as possible in every regard except the treatment that they receive. As will be seen in later chapters, this allows any difference in response between the treatment groups to be ascribed to the treatment they received.

Randomization is also important in nonclinical studies. Treatments should be assigned at random whether the experimental units are humans, animals, or test tubes. As Machin and Campbell (2005) noted, "Medical investigators often appreciate the effect that biological variation has in patients, but overlook or underestimate its presence in the laboratory."

Randomization in clinical trials is likely to make the weights of subjects in the treatments, on average, fairly similar. In nonclinical studies involving animals, where weight may be a particularly salient factor, it is possible to go one step further. Following randomization, the animals in each treatment group can be weighed and the groups compared. Statistical tests (examining homogeneity of variance and testing for a statistically significant difference in weight between the groups) can be conducted, and if the groups are not as similar as the researcher would like, the animals are rerandomized. This process can be repeated in an iterative manner until the researcher is satisfied that the treatment groups are sufficiently similar, as determined by a prespecified statistical criterion. This process is called censored randomization (Gad, 2006).

Part III

Design, Methodology, and Analysis

5

Design and Methodology in Clinical Trials

5.1 Introduction

Study design is the first component of an overall research process that, ideally, is integrated and seamless. In a real sense, separate discussions of design, methodology, and analysis impose artificial divisions on a process whose very nature is interactive and integrative. However, there is sometimes benefit in looking at components separately, since discussions can temporarily focus on one or two of them before illustrating the interrelatedness of all three. This chapter focuses on design and methodology.

Each study in a clinical development program addresses one or more research questions. Refining good research questions is critical to the potential success of all studies, since they suggest how the study needs to be designed to provide the information that will answer these questions. Choosing the best study design to answer the research question(s) is therefore critical. Good methodology is then necessary to obtain optimum quality data.

5.2 Design

The majority of discussions in this book focus on a simple study design used in clinical trials. This design can be described by a collection of terms with which you will become very familiar: It is a randomized, double-blind, concurrently controlled, parallel group trial. This design includes a treatment group, subjects receiving the drug under investigation, and a concurrent control group. The control group used most frequently in this book's examples is a group of subjects who take part in the trial at the same time as the drug treatment group (hence the term "concurrently" in the trial's name) and receive a placebo, a treatment that does not have any pharmacological activity. This group is referred to as the placebo treatment group. While other arrangements can certainly be used, the points made in our discussions will provide a solid overall understanding of clinical trial design.

5.3 Methodology

Experimental methodology is concerned with all aspects of the implementation and conduct of a study. Its goal is to govern the conduct of the study such that optimum quality data are acquired. To enable subsequent data analysis and interpretation to provide the best answer to the research question of interest, the data acquired must be of optimum quality. The most sophisticated and computationally perfect

New Drug Development: Design, Methodology, and Analysis. By J. Rick Turner

analysis will not yield optimal answers if the data being analyzed are of less than optimal quality. This statement sounds intuitively obvious and may seem almost superfluous. However, it is essential that methodological considerations receive constant vigilance in studies of even the shortest duration and in clinical trials that can last several years.

5.4 ETHICAL ASPECTS OF DESIGN AND METHODOLOGY

Correct design is absolutely essential from a scientific perspective when conducting clinical trials. Conducting a study whose design cannot lead to meaningful analysis of the data acquired cannot provide any meaningful information about the investigational drug. Such a study would be a colossal waste of time, human resources, and money. It would also be unethical.

Employment of human subjects in clinical trials is a sacrosanct undertaking. Subjects participate voluntarily, and they have every expectation that their welfare during the trial is of supreme importance to the researchers conducting the study. They also have the legitimate expectation that their participation in the trial will help advance knowledge concerning the experimental drug. If the design does not permit the research question to be addressed, that expectation is not fulfilled.

Extending this obligation to everyone involved in collecting and managing data, supreme care is needed at every stage so that optimum quality data are collected. Everyone involved in the execution of a trial needs to remain aware of this throughout the trial. Good study design coupled with poor methodology cannot produce optimum quality data: Neither can poor design and good methodology. Therefore, everyone involved in study design and methodology has an obligation to the subjects in a trial to make it possible for their participation to provide optimum quality data. If this is not done, some subjects have been exposed to the investigational drug unnecessarily, and therefore the benefit/risk balance is completely tilted in the risk direction.

5.5 STUDY DESIGN IN DRUG CLINICAL TRIALS

There are two fundamental types of study design: experimental and nonexperimental (Piantadosi, 2005). Piantadosi defines an experiment as a series of observations made under conditions in which the influences of interest are controlled by the research scientist. This book deals largely with experimental studies. In nonexperimental studies, the research scientist collects observations but does not exert control over the influences of interest. Nonexperimental studies are often called "observational" studies, but this term is inaccurate; it does not definitively distinguish between nonexperimental studies and experimental studies, in which observations are also made. Some nonexperimental study designs are discussed in Chapter 13.

It should be noted here that the term "nonexperimental" is not a relative quality judgment compared with "experimental." This nomenclature simply distinguishes methodological approaches. In some cases, nonexperimental studies are the only type of medical study that can legitimately be used. If one wishes to examine the potentially negative health impact of a specific influence, such as exposure to nicotine via smoking cigarettes or living close to an environmental toxin, it is not appropriate for the research scientist to exert control over the influence of interest by asking some individuals to smoke or to live in a certain location. Rather, the research scientist makes use of naturally occurring cases of individuals who have and have not smoked and individuals who live close to and far from an environmental toxin to examine a potential relationship between the influence of interest and a specific health outcome.

Piantadosi (2005) defined a clinical trial as an experiment that tests a medical treatment on human subjects. A common research question in drug clinical trials that are conducted in the later phases of a clinical development program is: Does a new drug under development have a beneficial therapeutic effect? To answer this question adequately, the therapeutic effect of the new drug needs to be compared with the therapeutic effect of something else. That is, a comparator treatment is needed. Such trials are called controlled trials. There are two fundamental approaches to providing a comparator treatment for this purpose. One is to employ a placebo. In this case, the terms "placebo control" and "placebo treatment" groups are typically used. This book focuses on this approach. It employs an ongoing example of testing a new drug with potential antihypertensive properties against a placebo. The second approach is to employ another drug. In this case, the drug chosen is one that is already known to demonstrate efficacy in treating (or preventing) the disease or condition for which the new drug is being developed. In this case, the terms "active control" and "active/control treatment" groups are typically used. This approach is not discussed to a large extent in this book, but it does feature in two study designs discussed in Chapter 11, i.e., equivalence and noninferiority trials. It is therefore appropriate here to note one particular aspect of active control trials that needs careful attention.

Demonstrating the therapeutic benefit of a new drug via the employment of an active controlled study, i.e., a study in which an active control is used as the comparator, requires assurance that the active control was actually efficacious in the study. If the active control is not efficacious (superior to placebo), it is quite possible that the new drug, even though it produced a numerically greater effect, was not efficacious either. Providing this assurance is the aspect of active control designs that requires careful attention. One way to provide this assurance directly would be to use a study design in which a placebo treatment group is also included. This three-group study design facilitates comparison of the active control directly against the placebo, which can provide evidence that it was indeed efficacious in this particular trial. However, if there is a very good expectation that this would be the case, this design is likely unethical, since a state of clinical equipoise would not exist between the active control and the placebo: As noted in Section 1.8.1, individuals agree to participate in a clinical trial with the understanding that all of the treatments in the trial are assumed to be of equal value. Therefore, if there is a very good expectation that the active control would show superiority to placebo, a placebo treatment group should not be included: However, acceptable demonstration of this "very good expectation" is then appropriate. One method of providing this acceptable demonstration might be to evaluate the literature concerning the active control. If it can be seen that the active control is "almost always" superior to placebo, it might well be acceptable to assume that, had a placebo control group been included in this trial, the active control would have been superior. Therefore, it is acceptable to conclude that, if the test drug produces a similar therapeutic effect as the active control (and "similar" requires a precise set of rules in each case: see Chapter 11), the test drug would also have been superior to placebo. (See ICH Guideline E10, Choice of Control Group and Related Issues in Clinical Trials, for additional discussion.)

Two commonly employed designs in new drug development are the parallel group design and the cross-over design. These are described here in their basic forms, in which there are just two treatment groups, the drug treatment group and a control treatment group. Virtually all discussion of clinical trial design in this book will focus on designs in which just two treatment groups are employed. There are two reasons behind this decision. First, these simple designs are very informative. Second, this strategy permits the central topics of this book to be illustrated and described in a straightforward manner. An understanding and working knowledge of designs employing two treatment groups will enable you to understand the fundamentals of more complex designs very easily. Both of these designs are flexible and can be readily adapted to provide additional information in more complex formats.

5.5.1 The Parallel Group Design

In the parallel group design, one group of subjects is administered the drug and a second group of subjects is administered the control compound. These groups are called the drug treatment group and the control treatment group, respectively. The influence of interest, the pharmacological effect of the drug under investigation, is therefore under the research scientist's control, since a certain identified group of subjects receive the drug treatment while another identified group of subjects receive the control treatment. If due attention is paid to methodological and statistical considerations, especially to randomization, differential physiological responses between these treatment groups can be attributed to the difference between the drug and the control compound. Randomization is a process that facilitates the random and independent allocation of trial subjects to the different treatment groups (see Section 5.6.2).

5.5.2 The Cross-Over Design

In contrast to the parallel group design, in which a given individual receives only one of the two treatments, subjects in a cross-over trial receive both treatments during the course of the experiment. Senn (2002) defined a cross-over trial as one in which subjects are given sequences of treatments with the objective of studying differences between the individual treatments. A common and simple design is one in which half the subjects receive treatment A first and treatment B second, while the other half receive treatment B first followed by treatment A. A washout period in the middle is employed to ensure that all pharmacological activity of the first drug administered has finished by the time the second treatment is administered.

5.5.3 The Respective Advantages of the Parallel Group and Cross-Over Designs

The cross-over design has one considerable theoretical advantage over the parallel group design. Its nature is such that each subject receives both treatments, which means that each subject's response to one treatment can be compared directly with the same subject's response to the other treatment. This allows a within-subjects statistical analysis to be employed to analyze these data (see Section 7.7). Such analyses are relatively more powerful than between-subjects designs that are used in parallel group studies. The power of a statistical test is an important consideration in any experimental design (Jones, 2002). Generally, the power of a statistical test may be defined as "the probability that the Null Hypothesis is rejected when it is indeed false" (Jones, 2002). The null hypothesis, and its central role in hypothesis testing, is discussed in Chapter 7.

In contrast, the nature of the parallel group design is such that each subject receives only one treatment. Comparison of treatments requires comparing the responses of one group of individuals (the drug treatment group) with those of the second group of individuals (the control treatment group). The between-subjects statistical analysis that must be employed to analyze these data (see Section 7.6) is relatively less powerful than the within-subjects analysis used for the cross-over trial.

However, practical considerations often make employment of a cross-over design impractical or impossible. Additionally, in some cases where a cross-over design would be possible, the length of treatment administration for each subject may mean that adoption of this design would be very expensive and therefore cost inefficient. Since this design requires that subjects receive one treatment first and then the other afterward, it takes at least twice as long to implement (depending on the length of the washout period) as a parallel group design.

5.5.4 Focus on the Parallel Group Design in This Book

We will focus on the parallel group design in this book, since it is a relatively simple and very common design in new drug development, and its use is well suited to illustrate the major points of interest. As noted, in many cases the control group of interest is a placebo treatment group. This is a common design employed in superiority trials, where the goal is to demonstrate that the investigational drug is safe and is superior in efficacy to the control treatment. In the equivalence trials and noninferiority trials discussed in Chapter 11, the control group of interest is a treatment group in which the subjects are administered an active comparator drug.

5.6 CENTRAL PRINCIPLES OF EXPERIMENTAL DESIGN IN CLINICAL TRIALS

The designs used in most clinical trials are actually relatively simple designs. Clinical trials are certainly complex, but this complexity is not a direct function of the nature of the designs employed, but the result of other factors such as "ethics, biology, logistics, and execution" (Piantadosi, 2005). Clinical trials embody the following fundamental principles of experimental design:

- Replication: more than one experimental unit (here, subjects) is used in each treatment group to estimate variability.
- Randomization: to ensure validity.
- Local control: performed to reduce experimental error.

More specifically in the context of clinical trials, proper design confers many advantages, including the following:

- Allows investigators to satisfy ethical considerations.
- Isolates the treatment effect from confounding influences.
- Minimizes and quantifies random error.
- Reduces selection bias and observer bias (nonrandom error).
- Increases the external validity of the trial.
- Simplifies and validates the accompanying statistical analyses.

We will consider replication, randomization, and local control in turn.

5.6.1 Replication

Clinical trials employ more than one subject in each treatment group. The reason for this is that there is considerable variation in how individuals respond to the administration of the same drug. It is therefore simply not possible to choose only one subject to receive the new drug and another to receive the placebo: There is no way of knowing how representative the subject's response to the drug is of the typical response of people in general. The need to include more than one person is a driving force behind all of the statistical approaches discussed.

5.6.2 Randomization

Randomization involves randomly assigning experimental subjects to one of the treatment groups so that the many potential influences that cannot be controlled for (e.g., height, weight) or cannot be determined by observation (e.g., specific metabolic pathway influences) are likely to be as frequent in one treatment group as they are in the other. Randomization occurs after a subject's eligibility for a clinical trial has been determined and before any experimental data are collected. The purpose of randomization is to facilitate the random assignment of subjects to different treatment groups with the intent of avoiding any selection bias in subject assignment. The process of randomization is facilitated by the generation of a randomization list. This list is generated (often by a random-number generator) in advance of recruiting the first subject. The randomization list is generated under the direction of the trial statistician. To maintain confidentiality, the list is not released to the trial statistician until the completion of the study.

As will be seen in Chapter 7, inferential statistics requires the random assignment of subjects to different treatment groups to allow differences in drug responses between treatment groups to be connected to the treatments administered. Randomization means that other potential sources of influence on the data have been randomly allocated to each treatment group. That is, subjects have an independent (and usually, but not necessarily, equal) chance of receiving either the investigational drug or control treatment. The phrase "usually, but not necessarily, equal" is used here because, while subjects are typically randomized to two treatment groups in a 1:1 ratio, leading to the same number of subjects randomized to each group, it is possible to use other randomization ratios. For example, a ratio of 2:1 for treatment versus placebo would mean that two thirds of the subjects would be randomized to the treatment group and one third to the placebo group. Such a ratio has two implications. First, the statistical power to detect a difference between the groups is not as high as it would be if the number of subjects in each group were equal (a point made also in the next section). On the other hand, more safety data concerning the new drug will be gained, since two-thirds of the total number of subjects in the study will receive this treatment, instead of one-half. In some cases, the sponsor will be willing to settle for less statistical power to gain the advantage of collecting more safety data.

The goal of randomization is to eliminate bias (see also Berger, 2005). This includes subject bias based on their knowledge of which treatment group they have been assigned to and investigator bias. Investigator bias is eliminated by preventing investigators from deliberately assigning patients to one treatment group or the other. Two possible unconscious or conscious biases on the part of the investigators that are thus removed are an inclination to place less healthy subjects in the treatment group receiving the drug they believe to be most beneficial and an inclination to place the more healthy subjects in the investigational drug group to demonstrate its superiority.

Simple randomization.

Kay (2005) highlighted several methods of randomization, including simple randomization, block randomization, and stratified randomization. Simple randomization involves assigning treatments to subjects in a completely random way. While this strategy is attractively simple, it is not advisable in the case of small trials. In the example of a trial involving 30 subjects randomized to two treatment groups, the probability of a 15–15 split, the most powerful from a statistical analysis point of view, is only 0.144, while the probability of a split of 11–19 or even more unbalanced is 0.20 (Kay, 2005). While 30 subjects is a small number that is used for illustrative purposes here, some sponsors advocate not using simple randomization schedules in trials with less than 200 participants: In such trials the stratified randomization approach, discussed shortly, is recommended (Ascione, 2001).

Block randomization.

Block randomization (sometimes called permuted blocked randomization) addresses the issue of potential unequal distribution of subjects to the treatment groups in a simple randomization schedule by guaranteeing that the numbers of subjects allocated to each treatment are equal at the end of randomization for every block of subjects. Blocks of various sizes can be chosen, and for each block there will be a specified number of permutations for how the subjects in that block can be equally allocated to the treatment groups. The most advantageous block size for a given trial depends on the number of treatments involved (the number of treatment arms) and the numbers of subjects that participating investigative sites can recruit.

Stratified randomization.

Stratified randomization adds another degree of sophistication. If there are readily identifiable characteristics, or prognostic factors, in the subject sample for which we might want to see fairly equitable distribution in the treatment groups, the randomization schedule can address this. Examples of these factors are severity of disease, high and low risk of a specified outcome, gender, and age. In this case, there needs to be a reason for the stratification, perhaps based on information obtained earlier in the drug development program. Also, it is advisable not to have too many strata, since obtaining equitable subject randomization across all strata can become increasingly difficult as the number of specified strata increases (Kay, 2005).

Cluster randomization.

In some circumstances, instead of randomly assigning individuals to treatment conditions, it is informative to randomly assign groups of individuals to these conditions (Campbell et al., 2004). Examples of these groups are families and medical practices. The designs of these trials are called cluster randomized trials. Compared with trials in which individual subjects are randomized, these trials are more complex to design, conduct, and analyze. Cluster randomized trials are considered briefly again in Section 13.6.3 in the context of reporting the results of these clinical trials.

Additional statistical steps to address randomization issues.

In parallel group designs, randomization is the most likely effective strategy to produce treatment groups with similar characteristics. Baseline characteristics should ideally be distributed equally, but this is not actually guaranteed by the process of randomization. This simple realization has two corollaries. First, before describing the results of a trial, baseline characteristics are described using descriptive statistics (see Chapter 10). This strategy allows a visual inspection of any imbalance in this regard. Second, a statistical technique called analysis of covariance (ANCOVA) can be used to statistically control for any baseline imbalances that may occur by chance despite randomization (see Chapter 11).

Ethical concerns regarding randomization.

Ascione (2001) addressed ethical concerns in the use of randomization in clinical trials. Clinicians and other health care professionals have an obligation to provide patients with the best care that they can: It is unethical for them to do otherwise. Sometimes, arguments are expressed that randomized clinical trials are not ethical since half of the subjects in a randomized placebo-controlled trial will receive a placebo and not the investigational drug. The key counterargument here is that there is an important difference between the clinical care that must be given to a patient and the role of a subject in a clinical trial. At the time of a trial's conduct it is not known for certain whether the investigational drug is actually more effective than the placebo. The purpose of the clinical development program is to establish whether or not the drug is effective. Indeed, by far the best way to establish the drug's efficacy is to conduct a randomized controlled trial. Once established, clinicians can use this information in determining the appropriate treatment for their patients.

There are well-established guidelines and procedures that enable investigators to largely overcome any ethical objections to the conduct of randomized trials. Fundamental to these procedures is the concept of informed consent. Subjects who take part in clinical trials must be provided with full information about the trial via an informed consent form (ICF) and the accompanying explanations and answers to all of the subjects' questions provided by the investigator. Subject participation is therefore undertaken in an informed and voluntary manner. In trials where subjects are not denied access to therapy that could alter survival or prevent irreversible injury, subjects participate in this research for the "greater good," acknowledging that their participation may help to produce compelling evidence that an investigational drug is indeed safe and effective. Once this is known, many patients may benefit from this finding, including subjects that received the investigational drug during the trial and are prescribed it later and also subjects with the same disease or condition that participated in the trial and received the placebo.

5.6.3 Local Control

Tight control on all aspects of methodology, e.g., the manner in which the treatments are administered, the manner in which measurements are made, and the apparatus used to make these measurements, must be exercised at all investigative sites. For example, it is not appropriate that blood pressures for all subjects in one treatment group are measured using one strategy and measuring device while blood pressures for all subjects in the other treatment group are measured differently. Every aspect of blood pressure measurement should be as uniform as possible for all subjects in the trial. (See Section 5.12 for a discussion of blood pressure.)

Environmental conditions should also be controlled as much as possible. Taking measurements and evaluating some subjects in relatively cold conditions and others in a relatively warmer environment are not recommended. Taking this example further, and considering factors such as ease of access to the investigative site and the general atmosphere (relaxed, frenetic) of the site and its investigators, it is not appropriate to have all subjects in one treatment group enrolled at one investigative site and all subjects in the other treatment group enrolled at a different site. The strategy of randomization can be used to preclude this.

5.6.4 Good Design Simplifies and Validates the Accompanying Analyses

As Piantadosi (2005) stated, "good designs are usually simple to analyze correctly (p. 129)." Good designs and good execution of the trial result in optimum quality data that can then be analyzed meaningfully. In contrast, poorly designed and executed studies yield less than optimum quality data, and some shortcomings of such trials cannot be corrected for by analysis. One of these shortcomings is systematic error, e.g., selection bias. A second is lack of precision in the estimate of the treatment effect, the difference between the mean effect in the drug group and the mean effect in the control group. High precision comes from employing an adequate sample size.

5.6.5 Sample-Size Estimation

Sample-size estimation is a critical part of the design of clinical trials, and, like all design issues, this must be addressed in the study protocol before the study commences. It may therefore seem logical to place discussion of sample-size estimation in this chapter along with the discussions of other design issues. However, placement of this vital topic raises an interesting conundrum. Meaningful consideration of sample-size estimation requires a certain understanding of statistical theory and statistical applications, topics that are addressed in Chapters 6–8. Therefore, while sample-size estimation is a vital part of study design, it is discussed in Chapter 9. At that point, you will have been introduced to the fundamentals of Statistics and statistical analysis and the concepts of statistical significance and clinical significance.

5.7 THE CLINICAL STUDY PROTOCOL

The study protocol is "the most important document in clinical trials, since it ensures the quality and integrity of the clinical investigation in terms of its planning, execution, conduct, and the analysis of the data" (Chow and Chang, 2007). The study protocol is a comprehensive plan of action that contains information concerning the goals of the study, details of subject recruitment, details of safety monitoring, and all aspects of design, methodology, and analysis. Input is therefore required, for example, from clinical scientists, medical safety officers, study managers, data managers, and statisticians. Consequently, while one clinical scientist or medical writer may take primary responsibility for its preparation, many members of the study team make critical contributions to it.

Buncher and Tsay (2006a) listed just some of the detailed requirements of a study protocol:

- Primary and secondary objectives. These are stated as precisely as possible.
- Measures of efficacy. The criteria to be used to determine efficacy are provided.
- Statistical analysis. The precise analytical strategy needs to be detailed, here and/or in an associated statistical analysis plan.
- Diagnosis of the disease or condition. When subjects are required to have the disease or condition for which the drug is intended, precise diagnostic criteria are provided.
- Inclusion and exclusion criteria. These provide detailed criteria for subject eligibility for participation in the trial (see Section 5.7.1).
- Clinical and laboratory procedures. Full details of the nature and timing of all procedures and tests are provided.
- Drug treatment schedule. Route of administration, dosage, and dosing regimen are detailed. This information is also provided for the control treatment.

5.7.1 Inclusion and Exclusion Criteria

Inclusion and exclusion criteria are a very important component of clinical trials. A study's inclusion and exclusion criteria govern the subjects who may be admitted to the study. Criteria for inclusion in the study may include items such as the following:

- Reliable evidence of a diagnosis of the disease or condition of interest.
- A specified age range.
- Willingness to take measures to prevent becoming pregnant during the course of treatment.

Criteria for exclusion from the study may include items such as the following:

- Taking certain medications for other reasons and which cannot safely be stopped during the trial.
- Participation in another clinical trial within so many months prior to the commencement of this study.
- Liver or kidney disease.

While inclusion and exclusion criteria are typically provided in two separate lists in regulatory documentation, exclusion criteria can be regarded as further refinements of the inclusion criteria. Meeting all the inclusion criteria allows a subject to be considered as a study participant, while not meeting any exclusion criteria is also necessary to allow the subject to become a participant. In the language of mathematics, meeting the stated inclusion criteria is necessary but not sufficient to gain entry to the study.

Inclusion and exclusion criteria strictly define the nature of the subject sample that participates in a clinical trial. Accordingly, they also strictly define the study population to which statistical inferences may be made (see Chapter 7 for discussion of statistical inference). For now, this statement can be expressed as follows: The inclusion and exclusion criteria strictly define the study population to whom the results of the clinical trial can reasonably be generalized. This study population may or may not be a good representation of the entire population of patients with the disease or condition of interest. Chapter 11 provides more detailed discussion of the implications of this statement. (See also www.clinicaltrials.gov for examples of inclusion and exclusion criteria in clinical trials.)

5.7.2 The Primary Objective

It is a very good idea to have a clear, concise, unambiguous protocol that is as short as possible while maintaining its scientific integrity. However, this ideal is not always achieved. Buncher and Tsay (2006a) noted that one dilemma faced by writers of study protocols is "the challenge to maintain a balance between brevity and completeness." All necessary procedural information must be included to allow the principal investigators and their coinvestigators and staff at each study site (investigational site) to implement the protocol exactly as intended. However, as the length of the protocol increases, it is unfortunately likely that the chances of it being read and complied with in its entirety decrease commensurately after a certain point. This means that investigator-related protocol violations become more likely, which in turn impacts statistical analyses that are conducted following the study (see Section 11.2.2 for discussion of the per-protocol study population). Clarity and conciseness are therefore very beneficial characteristics of the protocol.

A major reason that protocols can be (too) lengthy is that they can contain far more objectives than are actually necessary to address the goals of the particular study. As a development program proceeds, later studies often build on earlier studies, and this progression in itself is meaningful and important. However, it can be the case that the list of objectives increases excessively over time because objectives that were extremely pertinent in earlier studies are not removed from current protocols. This is undesirable for two reasons. First, there is a clear scientific and statistical benefit to having just one or maybe two primary objectives (see Section 11.4.1). Second, when there is an excess of objectives listed, methodological details relevant to these extra objectives need to be included in the protocol. This can add considerable and unnecessary length to the protocol.

Derenzo and Moss (2006) provided a detailed discussion of clinical research protocols, and readers are directed to their book.

5.8 COLLECTING DATA: THE CASE REPORT FORM

Case report forms (CRFs) are used throughout clinical trials to record data collected during a trial. They record all of the information specified in the protocol for each subject (all data recorded on the CRF must be verifiable from original source documentation). While the traditional paper CRF format is still used, electronic data collection is becoming more common. Voorhees and Scheipeter (2005) discussed CRF development in detail, highlighting some of the fundamental aspects of their purpose, design, and nature:

- Well-designed CRFs capture all essential scientific and regulatory information and do not capture information that is not needed. Collected data include those related to study endpoints, adverse events (AEs), potential confounding influences, and protocol compliance.
- Their design benefits considerably from involvement by sponsors who record information on them and statisticians who will eventually be analyzing the data.
- They should be clear, easy to read, and able to be completed quickly and efficiently and capture data unambiguously.

Good (2006) noted some other points:

- Design your CRFs accordingly. Do not start by simply deciding to use the data collection forms that were used in previous studies. If there are some questions on previous forms that address the collection of data you need, can those questions be improved?
- Create forms that are designed to collect the data you need and only the data

you need. That is, create data collection forms that provide data that will address the objectives of the study and only those objectives. Collecting additional data is unnecessarily wasteful of time, money, and resources.

Prokscha (2007) commented that a cross-functional team is needed to design a CRF that is clear and easily completed by the investigators, is efficient for data management processes, facilitates statistical analysis appropriately, and can therefore provide data that can allow decisions to be made concerning the safety and efficacy of the drug.

5.9 CLINICAL DATA MANAGEMENT

It is noted several times in this book that the goal of experimental methodology is to provide optimum quality data for subsequent statistical analysis. This is true, but there is also a very important intermediary between data acquisition and data analysis; this is the field of clinical data management. In many cases, Data Management and Statistics fall under the same division within a company, and in some cases these tasks are handled by different divisions. Whichever is the case, it is vital to have statisticians involved in all discussions regarding database development and use.

Data analysis is typically conducted using files of data collected in a clinical trial. These files are typically contained in databases. It is of critical importance that the data collected from all sources are accurately captured in the database. A brief list of such data includes subject identifiers (rather than their names), age, height, weight, questionnaire data concerning a multitude of topics, physiological measurements made before, during, and possibly after the treatment period, adverse events reported, and laboratory data representing the results of assays made on blood samples taken from subjects at many points during the trial.

Ensuring that all of these data are in the database correctly is an enormous task, and one that is covered in this chapter only briefly. Section 10.14 provides a brief discussion of safety databases. For more detailed discussions, see Prokscha (2007).

5.9.1 The Data Management Plan

A data management plan for a clinical trial should be written along with the study protocol and the statistical analysis plan before the study commences. It identifies the documentation that will be produced as a result of all of the data collected during the conduct of the trial, who will be responsible for collecting the data, and which of the sponsor's documents (standard operating procedures or guidelines) will govern these activities. Prokscha (2007) listed topics that are covered by a data management plan, including:

- Design of the CRF.
- Entering data once collected.
- Cleaning the data.
- Managing laboratory data (see Section 10.15 for additional discussion).
- Serious adverse event (SAE) data handling (see Section 10.14.2 for additional discussion).
- Creating reports of data and transferring data.
- Quality assurance processes that will be implemented to ensure that all data management procedures are compliant with regulatory governance.

The quality assurance component is vital. Quality assurance (QA) is a process that involves the prevention, detection, and correction of errors or problems, and quality control (QC) is a check of the process (Prokscha, 2007). The data stored in the database need to be complete and accurate. Processes that check data and correct them (i.e., make a change to the database) where necessary need to be documented, and all corrections need to be documented in an audit trail such that a later audit can reveal exactly how the final database was created.

5.9.2 Electronic Data Capture

It is helpful to utilize electronic data capture when possible. Computer-assisted data entry, or electronic data capture, at the time of the subject's clinic visit or procedure makes the data entry process quicker and less susceptible to error. It also offers the chance to monitor data collection in a timely manner as the clinical trial progresses, which facilitates the opportunity to detect trends toward poor quality or unexpected data that may be the result of the investigator site failing to adhere to the protocol. Early detection and correction are much preferable to the alternative.

5.9.3 Database Development

Having collected optimal quality data, first-rate data management is also critical. Many data that are collected can now be fed directly from the measuring instrument to computer databases, thereby avoiding the potential of human data entry error. However, this is not universally true. Therefore, careful strategies have been developed to scrutinize data as they are entered and once they are in the database. The "double-entry method" requires that each data set be entered twice (usually by two operators) and these entries compared by a computer for any discrepancies. This method operates on the model that two identical errors are probabilistically very unlikely, and that every time the two entries match the data are correct. In contrast, dissimilar entries are identified, the source (original) data located, and the correct data point entry confirmed.

A tremendous amount of measurements and evaluations are made in clinical trials. To facilitate the eventual statistical analysis of these data, recording and maintaining them are extremely important. Database development, implementation, and maintenance therefore require considerable attention. The goals of a formal database are to store data in a manner that facilitates prompt retrieval while not diminishing their security or integrity (Mulvihill et al, 2005).

There are several types of database models. Clinical research typically utilizes one of two types, the flat file type database or the relational database. Each has its advantages and disadvantages, and these will be considered by data managers before they decide which type to employ. The flat file database model is simple but restrictive, and it becomes less easy to use as the amount of data stored increases. This model can also lead to data redundancy (the same information, e.g., a subject's name, being entered multiple times) and consequently to potential errors (misspelling of the subject's name on some of these occasions). This model often works well for relatively small databases. Relational databases are more flexible, but they can be complex, and careful initial work needs to be done. This work involves initial logical modeling of the database. The defining feature of a relational database is that data are stored in tables, and these tables can be related to each other. This reduces data redundancy. Subject names in one table, for example, can be related to their heights in another table, their baseline blood pressure in another table, and so on, thereby eliminating the need to store names with each individual set of measurements. Since these databases can contain huge amounts of tables, use of one of several commercially available relational database management systems (RDBMSs) is typical. Regardless of the type of database employed, care must be taken in data entry and in protecting the integrity, and in many cases the security, of the data (Mulvihill et al., 2005).

This last point is very important in two ways. First, throughout this book, the importance of optimum quality data is emphasized many times. In most cases, this comment is associated with acquiring the data, for example, measuring blood pressure as accurately as possible. However, since all of these data are entered into databases, data entry must be accurate: A correct measurement that is stored incorrectly immediately lessens the quality of the overall data. Sometimes data are transferred from a measurement device electronically to the database, and sometimes data are manually entered into the database. Procedures to ensure accuracy, correctness, and completeness of data transfer are an essential part of data recording and management. Second, the storage of sensitive data (personal, medical) and proprietary data requires additional considerations to ensure that these data do not become accessible and available to unauthorized users.

5.10 MONITORING CLINICAL TRIALS

Since clinical trials can be conducted at multiple investigative sites (quite possibly in several countries) and can last for several years, it is essential for the acquisition of optimum quality data that the progress of the trial is monitored. Monitoring is typically performed by individuals with titles such as clinical research associates (CRAs), clinical research monitors (CRMs), and medical monitors. Monitors have responsibilities before the trial starts and throughout its implementation. Preliminary visits to sites enable relationships with investigators and their colleagues to be established and training to be conducted. Also before the trial commences, the monitor will go through an extensive pretrial checklist to ensure, for example, that initial supplies of the drugs (the test drug and the placebo or active comparator drug) have arrived, electronic data capture equipment is installed and tested, and informed consent forms and procedural manuals are available. Among the issues where monitoring is essential are recruiting and retaining subjects and investigators, checking on protocol compliance, performing a quality control function, evaluating subject adherence to the trial's treatment regimens, and limiting adverse events (Good, 2006).

One of the main quality control functions of the monitor is oversight of data collection in CRFs. The responsibilities of the monitor here include checking on investigators' compliance with the protocol, subject safety, and thorough and complete reporting of all AEs.

5.11 PROJECT MANAGEMENT

Project management is a critical overall aspect of conducting clinical trials, and, while it is not discussed in detail here, its importance in the success of a clinical trial cannot be overstated. Cook (2004) discussed various components of project management, including goals, budgets, timelines, resources, measurement, communication, and training. All of these components must be successfully planned and implemented. In addition, project managers must conduct their work against a backdrop of tremendous scientific, technical, and financial risks (see Robinson and Cook, 2005). Readers are referred to these sources for more details (see also Krupa, 2006).

5.12 BLOOD PRESSURE AND BLOOD PRESSURE MEASUREMENT

Throughout this book, a common therapeutic area is used for most aspects of design, methodology, and analysis discussed. Many texts utilize real data from various therapeutic areas to make individual points, and this strategy works extremely well in many cases. However, the goal of this book is to provide a fundamental conceptual knowledge and understanding of design, methodology, and analysis in new drug development, and a uniformity of approach with regard to the therapeutic area being discussed provides one less distraction. The therapeutic area discussed is high blood pressure, or hypertension, and discussions focus on the development of a new drug with antihypertensive properties.

5.12.1 Surrogate Endpoints

Two major clinical endpoints of disease are morbidity and mortality, and medical intervention, including drug therapy, is concerned with reducing both. As Oliver and Webb (2003) observed, however, assessing whether a drug has positive effects on morbidity and mortality can be time-consuming and costly. Therefore, rather than focus on outcomes that are directly relevant to patients, clinical trials often substitute surrogate endpoints for clinical endpoints and assess these surrogate endpoints in the participating subjects.

Machin and Campbell (2005) defined a surrogate endpoint as "a biomarker (or other indicator) that is intended to substitute for an (often) clinical endpoint and predict its behavior." The authors also noted that, if a surrogate endpoint is to be used, there is a very important need to ensure that it is "an appropriate surrogate for the (true) endpoint of concern." An important characteristic of a surrogate endpoint is biological plausibility. There should be evidence that the surrogate endpoint is on the causal pathway to the clinical endpoint of interest. A detailed knowledge and understanding of the pathophysiology of the disease or condition of clinical interest coupled with similar knowledge of the drug's mechanism of action can provide a solid basis for believing that the drug will be beneficial. Another important characteristic is that the surrogate endpoint predicts the clinical endpoint consistently and independently (Oliver and Webb, 2003).

Surrogate endpoints are particularly useful in cases where the clinical endpoints occur after long periods. This is particularly relevant to cardiovascular disease. High blood pressure is a well-established cardiovascular surrogate endpoint; it is well established that chronic high blood pressure is causative of cardiovascular and cerebrovascular events. Kannel and Sorlie (1975) commented on data from the Framingham Heart Study, a major prospective cardiovascular study of over 5,000 individuals:

> Compared to "normotensives," "hypertensive" persons develop a marked excess of the major cardiovascular diseases. In the age group 45-74, they develop at least twice as much occlusive peripheral artery disease, about three times as much coronary disease, more than four times as much congestive [heart] failure and over seven times the incidence of brain infarction as normotensives.

Given that around 50 million people in the United States and one billion people worldwide have high blood pressure, the development of antihypertensive drugs is of considerable interest (see Lednicer, 2007).

There are several advantages of using blood pressure assessment in this context (Oliver and Webb, 2003):

- Clinical trials can be run more efficiently, at lower cost, and in a shorter timeframe.
- The number of subjects needed to demonstrate an effect on a surrogate endpoint is likely considerably less than that needed to demonstrate an effect on the clinical endpoint of interest.
- Every person has a blood pressure, whereas only a subset will die or have a cardiovascular event in a period of a few years (a timeframe that can be monitored in a typical clinical trial).
- A drug's effect on a surrogate endpoint can be measured much sooner that its effect on the clinical endpoint of interest.

5.12.2 Arterial Blood Pressure

There is continuous pressure in the arteries to provide the driving force necessary to propel blood through the capillaries, where oxygen is given to body tissues and carbon dioxide collected for transport back to the lungs via the venous system. The level of pressure fluctuates during each cardiac cycle. Commonly cited healthy arterial blood pressure values for adults are a systolic blood pressure (SBP) value of 120 millimeters of mercury (mmHg) and a diastolic blood pressure (DBP) of 80 mmHg.

This unit of measurement is used because the pressure in the artery, if channeled to the bottom of a column of mercury, would cause the mercury to rise a certain number of millimeters in height. The first invasive methods of measuring blood pressure employed such a mercury column, and, given the fluctuation that occurs throughout each cardiac cycle, the height of the mercury varied throughout the cycle. While this invasive method is a very precise method of measurement, it is cumbersome and carries risks associated with all invasive procedures. A modified and noninvasive version of this procedure is therefore very practical. Such a procedure is used to measure blood pressure in current clinical settings each time a mercury sphygmomanometer is used.

The reason for the use of a mercury column is that mercury is considerably heavier than liquids such as water, which appears to be a much more convenient (and less toxic) option. Water could certainly be used theoretically, but, since it is approximately 13 times less heavy than mercury, the sphygmomanometer column would need to be 13 times as high. The height of ceilings in typical clinical settings and the difficulty of reading the level of the liquid at the heights that would be needed effectively preclude such an option (Turner, 1994).

Other blood pressure measuring devices are also used routinely.

5.12.3 Defining High Blood Pressure

The Seventh Report of the Joint National Committee on Prevention, Detection, Evaluation, and Treatment of High Blood Pressure (JNC 7: NIH, 2004) is a definitive publication concerning the treatment (behavioral and pharmacological) of high blood pressure. It provides the following blood pressure classifications for adult blood pressures:

- Normal: SBP < 120 mmHg and DBP < 80 mmHg.
- Prehypertension: SBP 120–139 mmHg or DBP 80–89 mmHg.
- Stage 1 hypertension: SBP 140–159 mmHg or DBP 90–99 mmHg.
- Stage 2 hypertension: SBP ≥ 160 mmHg or DBP ≥ 100 mmHg.

These classifications are related to management strategies for high blood pressure. This report is the first of the JNC's reports to use the term "prehypertension," a term introduced to signal the need for increased awareness and education among health care professionals and the general public to reduce blood pressure before it reaches the levels in the hypertensive categories. The relationship between blood pressure and risk of cardiovascular events is "continuous, consistent, and independent of other risk factors. The higher the BP, the greater is the chance of heart attack, heart failure, stroke, and kidney disease" (NIH, 2004). Thus, while the classifications provided are very useful for directing the management of blood pressure by clinicians, who have to make a decision to treat or not to treat a patient, it should be recognized that while a blood pressure of 135/85 mmHg falls in the prehypertensive classification, and therefore does not reach the Stage 1 hypertension classification, it carries a higher risk than lower pressures within the same classification.

5.12.4 Measuring Blood Pressure Change over Time

A clinical trial involving an antihypertensive drug requires assessing blood pressure change over time, which necessitates measurements at two time points or more. Imagine a clinical trial in which the treatment phase lasts 12 weeks. A baseline measurement is obtained for each subject before the start of the treatment phase, and a subsequent measurement taken at the end of the treatment phase. In practice, it is also likely that measurements will be taken at various specified intervals during the treatment phase.

The exact schedule of measurements is decided upon by the study team and governed by the study design and the study protocol. One hypothetical study may require that subjects return to the investigational site once a week throughout the treatment phase, while another may require that measurements are made at week 2, week 4, week 8, and week 12. Both of these schedules allow the examination of blood pressure change over time, with the former's more frequent measurements allowing a higher degree of resolution of this change. For ease of description throughout the book, just two blood pressure measurements will be considered, the baseline measurement and the end-of-treatment measurement. (The statistical methodology is also easier in this case: Dealing with multiple measurements during the treatment phase requires additional techniques to be employed.)

The use of a baseline measurement allows random subject-to-subject variation to be reduced to a certain degree. Imagine a scenario where only end-of-treatment measurements were made and imagine hypothetical data from two subjects, "subject A" who is in the drug treatment group, and "subject B" who is in the control treatment group. The end-of-treatment SBP measurement for subject A is 120 mmHg and the end-of-treatment SBP measurement for subject B is 110 mmHg. While no real clinical trial would ever involve only two participants, consideration of these hypothetical data is instructive in this context. Based only on these two end-of-treatment measurements, 12 weeks of treatment with the drug has resulted in a SBP of 120 mmHg, while 12 weeks of treatment with the control has resulted in a SBP of 110 mmHg, a lower value. Based on these data alone, it is understandable how the conclusion could be made that the control is "more effective" in lowering SBP since it resulted in a lower SBP reading at the end of 12 weeks of treatment.

The key to assessing the relative efficacy of the drug compared with the control compound lies in taking baselines readings and examining the change over time. Since individuals differ in their physiology and in their blood pressure readings, different individuals are very likely to have different baseline readings. Imagine now that subject A had a baseline SBP of 140 mmHg, while subject B had a baseline SBP of 114 mmHg. Across 12 weeks of treatment, subject A's SBP dropped 20 mmHg while subject B's blood pressure dropped 4 mmHg. The conclusion that could understandably be reached is now very different: The drug is "more effective" in lowering SBP than the control since it resulted in a greater decrease in SBP across the 12 weeks of treatment. This conclusion is by far the more reasonable one. It is based on a strategy that takes into account that some individuals will have higher baseline readings than others and that the best way to evaluate the effect of the drug versus the control is to take into account both the baseline and the end-of-treatment measurements.

6

STATISTICAL ANALYSIS

6.1 INTRODUCTION

It was noted in Chapter 1 that, in the present context, Statistics can be thought of as an integrated discipline that includes several steps:

- Identifying a research question that needs to be answered.
- Deciding upon the design of the study, the methodology that will be employed, and the numerical information (data) that will be collected.
- Presenting the design, methodology, and data to be collected in a study protocol. This study protocol specifies the manner of data collection and addresses all methodological considerations necessary to ensure the collection of optimum quality data for subsequent statistical analysis.
- Identifying the statistical techniques that will be used to describe and analyze the data in an associated statistical analysis plan, which should be written in conjunction with the study protocol.
- Describing and analyzing the data. This includes analyzing the variation in the data to see if there is compelling evidence of systematic variation in the outcome variable of interest (usually "change in SBP" in this book) that is associated with the drug treatment administered and interpreting the numerical results obtained in the context of the study's research question.
- Presenting the results of a clinical study to a regulatory agency in a clinical study report, and, where appropriate, presenting the results to the clinical community in journal publications.

More succinctly, the ultimate goal of Statistics in the context of new drug development is to provide optimum quality research data and to determine, in a widely accepted manner whether or not there is acceptable evidence (i.e., acceptable to a regulatory agency) that the drug under investigation is safe and effective. If there is acceptable evidence, the drug will be approved for marketing and become available for prescription by clinicians when treating their patients.

This chapter introduces basic concepts in statistical analysis that are of relevance to describing and analyzing the data that are collected in clinical trials, the hallmark of new drug development. (Statistical analysis in nonclinical studies was addressed earlier in Chapter 4.) This chapter therefore sets the scene for more detailed discussion of the determination of statistical significance via the process of hypothesis testing in Chapter 7, evaluation of clinical significance via the calculation of confidence intervals in Chapter 8, and discussions of adaptive designs and of noninferiority/equivalence trials in Chapter 11.

New Drug Development: Design, Methodology, and Analysis. By J. Rick Turner

6.2 Types of Clinical Data

Before discussing how clinical data are described and analyzed, it is helpful to introduce several categories of data. Data are numerical representations of information, and different forms of numerical information have different characteristics that permit (or do not permit) certain analyses to be conducted on them. In clinical research, the term "variable" is often used when describing data for a particular characteristic of interest, since values for participants in a clinical trial will vary from one individual to another. Clinical data can fall within several categories, including numerical (continuous and discrete) data and categorical (ordinal and nominal) data.

6.2.1 Numerical Variables

Numerical variables can either be continuous or discrete. Continuous variables are measured on a continuous, uninterrupted scale and can take any value on that scale. For example, height, weight, blood pressure, and heart rate are continuous variables. Depending on how accurately we want (or are able) to measure these variables, values containing one or more decimal points are certainly possible. In contrast, discrete variables can only take certain values, which are usually integers (whole numbers). The number of visits to an emergency room made by a person in one year is measured in whole numbers and is therefore a discrete variable. A subject's response to a questionnaire item that requires the choice of one of several specified levels (e.g., 1=mild pain, 2=medium pain, 3=severe pain) yields a discrete variable.

6.2.2 Categorical Variables

Many variables that are clinically useful fall into categories. Ethnicity is one example of categorical data often collected in clinical trials. Place of birth and blood type are also categorical values. All of these examples of categorical variables are called nominal variables: Each possibility in the categories (e.g., Caucasian, African American, Hispanic, etc.) has a unique name, but the possibilities are not ordered in any meaningful way. When a nominal variable can be placed into only one of two categories, the term "dichotomous," or "binary," is used. One particularly relevant example of this occurs in clinical trials in which subjects are randomized to one of two treatment groups, those receiving the active drug and those receiving the placebo. Treatment assignment is therefore a dichotomous variable on these occasions. Gender is another dichotomous variable. Survival data where the status of the subject is classified as "Alive or not alive twelve months after surgery" would also be dichotomous.

When the possibilities in a category are ordered in a meaningful way, the variable is called an ordinal variable. Even though the possibilities are nonnumerical, they can be arranged in a meaningful order. Socioeconomic level is one example which can be meaningfully ordered from the least to the most affluent. Categorization of an adverse event as mild, moderate, or severe is also possible in an ordered fashion.

It is possible to categorize continuous data into ordered categories. In this case, the data would then be considered as ordinal. An example is to divide subjects in a study into groups of those who are less than 30 years of age, those who are 30 years of age but less than 50 years of age, and those who are 50 years of age and older. If this is done, part of the unique information contained in each individual age is lost (both 35 years of age and 45 years of age, different values, are placed into the same category), but benefits of this categorization in certain circumstances may outweigh this decrease in informational richness.

6.2.3 Parametric Tests and Nonparametric Tests

The term "parametric test," or "analysis," is introduced in Section 6.2.4. In broad terms, statistical analyses can be placed into one of two categories, parametric tests and nonparametric tests. This book almost exclusively discusses parametric tests, but it should be noted here that nonparametric tests are also very valuable analyses in appropriate circumstances. As with the terms "experimental design" and "nonexperimental design" (recall Section 5.5), the term "nonparametric" is not a relative quality judgment compared with "parametric." This nomenclature simply differentiates statistical approaches. In circumstances where nonparametric analyses are appropriate, they are powerful tests.

6.2.4 Focus on Numerical Data in This Book

While all of the preceding types of data are of considerable use in the broad field of clinical research, attention in this book will focus on numerical and categorical data. These data are commonly used in new drug development, and they allow the book's major points to be well demonstrated. Several (nonexhaustive) examples of the kinds of data reported in a clinical study report (CSR) include the following. First, a summary/description of the subjects participating in a clinical study is typically the first part, the demographic data, of the Results section in a CSR. The total number of subjects participating, the numbers of men and women, and the numbers of subjects in each ethnic group are typically reported. These totals are also broken down by treatment group. In the section of a CSR that addresses safety results, the total numbers of various side effects or adverse events (AEs) such as headache, fatigue, and nausea are reported for each treatment group. In the Efficacy section, statistical analyses addressing the efficacy of the drug under investigation are reported (see Chapters 10 and 11).

As will be seen in Section 6.3, continuous data can be characterized by two useful parameters, the arithmetic mean and the standard deviation. These parameters permit the application of certain statistical analyses, which are therefore called parametric analyses (Katz, 2001). These analyses are commonly performed in randomized controlled trials. It should be noted here, however, that certain sets of continuous data, even though they can be characterized by a mean and a standard deviation, are analyzed using nonparametric methods if initial inspection of the data reveals that they are clearly not normally distributed. The phrase "normally distributed" has a specific and important meaning in Statistics: the Normal distribution is discussed in Section 6.6.

6.3 DESCRIPTIVE STATISTICS: SUMMARIZING DATA

Descriptive Statistics involves the presentation of summary statistics, which are concise yet meaningful summaries of large amounts of data. One category of descriptive statistics is the measurement of central tendency.

6.3.1 Measures of Central Tendency

One of the most commonly used measures of central tendency is the mean, more correctly (but rarely) called the arithmetic mean, a term that unambiguously distinguishes it from the geometric mean. While very informative in some circumstances, the geometric mean is less commonly used, and, in the absence of the prefix arithmetic or geometric, the default interpretation of the term "mean" is the arithmetic mean. This is the convention followed in the rest of this book. The mean of a set of data points is therefore defined as their sum divided by the total number of data points.

Two other common measures of central tendency are the mode and the median. The mode is the most frequently occurring value in a data set. The median is a value such that, when the data are arranged in order of magnitude, an equal numbers of data points lie above and below it. For any odd number of data points (e.g., 9), obtaining the median is straightforward (in this example it is the 5th number). For an even number of data points (e.g., 10), the mean of the middle two observations (in this case, the 5th and 6th numbers) is calculated. An advantage of the median is that, in comparison to the mean, its value is less influenced by outliers, i.e., values that are uncommonly far from the mean in any given set of numbers. (This advantage is shared by the geometric mean.)

Measures of central tendency provide an indication of the "location" of the data. For data measured on a scale of 1–100, a mean of 89 would suggest that the data are, in general, located closer to the top end of the scale than to the bottom end.

6.3.2 Measures of Dispersion About a Central Value

Another common category of descriptive statistics is the measure of dispersion of a set of data about a central value. The range is the arithmetic difference between the greatest (maximum) and the least (minimum) value in a data set. While this characteristic is easily calculated and is useful in initial inspections of data sets, the range, by definition, only uses two of the values in a data set to provide an assessment of the spread of the data points. In a large data set, most pieces of numerical information are therefore not used in the calculation of the range, and it is not known whether many data points lie close to the minimum, maximum, or mean or in any other distribution pattern.

Two more sophisticated measures of dispersion are variance and the standard deviation. These measures are intimately related to each other and take account of all the units of numerical information in a data set. The calculation of variance involves calculating the deviation of each data point from the mean of the data set and squaring these values. The process of squaring the deviation is mathematically necessary, but it creates the problem that the units of measurement of variance are not the same as the units of measurement of the original data. In the vast majority of cases, the data points in our studies are not simply numbers, but numerical representations of information measured in certain units. For example, an SBP measurement of "125" is actually a measurement of "125 mmHg." Since the calculation of variance involves squaring certain values, the variance of a set of blood pressure data points would actually be measured in "squared millimeters of mercury," a nonhelpful unit. Fortunately, this problem can be solved very simply by calculating the square root of the variance. The resulting value is called the standard deviation (SD), and the unit of measurement of the SD is the same as the unit of measurement of the original data points. The SD is a very commonly presented descriptor in clinical trials. It is usually presented in conjunction with the mean in the form "mean ± SD."

6.4 INFERENTIAL STATISTICS: HYPOTHESIS TESTING

6.4.1 The Search for "Compelling Evidence"

The domain of Inferential Statistics provides accepted methods of analyzing data that permit statements, at various levels of confidence, of the likely existence of systematic variation in that data set. Put another way, Inferential Statistics permits the determination of whether or not the data collected in a research study provide compelling evidence of a systematic influence on the data. In the context of this book, it permits the determination of whether or not there is compelling evidence that the drug under investigation lowers SBP and facilitates quantification of the degree of confidence present in this determination. (Historically, inferential statistics has been used to evaluate efficacy data, while discussion of safety data has been descriptive. This situation may change in the future: see Chapter 10.) Inferential statistics therefore examines the variation in the outcome variable of interest, i.e., change in SBP, to determine if there is compelling evidence of systematic variation caused by the drug under investigation.

The question that inferential statistics asks and answers, then, can be framed as such: Is there compelling evidence of systematic variation in our data? More specifically, it can be expressed as: Is there compelling evidence in the data that the drug under investigation tends to influence variation in change in SBP in a systematic manner? Before discussing how this question is answered, the concept of systematic variation is addressed.

6.4.2 Variation and Systematic Variation

In the physical sciences, the same operation done under the same conditions always produces the same result. In mathematics, there are accepted starting points (axioms) upon which the rest of the discipline is built. For example, it is fundamentally accepted that 1 + 1 = 2, 2 + 2 = 4, and so on. These axioms make all subsequent mathematical calculations possible, and guarantee that the same calculation performed on the same data always produces the same answer. In the biological sciences, including pharmaceutical and clinical sciences, this uniformity of outcome is conspicuously absent. The effects of the administration of the same pharmacological agent to the same individual on two separate occasions will almost certainly not yield identical results. Relatedly, administration of the same pharmacological agent to two individuals (even if dose-adjusted for weight) will not yield identical effects. In a large group of people, such as a group of subjects in a randomized controlled trial, there will typically be considerable variation in response. In clinical research, therefore, the variations of response in the drug treatment group and the placebo treatment group need to be represented by widely accepted quantitative measures.

Systematic variation refers to a pattern in the data that is due to an identifiable source of influence. If the changes in SBP observed for subjects in the drug treatment group vary in a systematic manner from the changes in SBP observed for subjects in the placebo treatment group, this systematic variation is attributed to the drug administered: Correct research methodology facilitates this attribution since it isolates the type of drug administered as the only influence that differs between the groups.

6.4.3 Between-Group Variation and Within-Group Variation

Two types of variation facilitate the evaluation of potential differential responses in two treatment groups. These are between-group variation and within-group variation. Statistical analyses compare these two types of variation as part of the calculations involved in looking for compelling evidence of systematic variation between the two groups of subjects. Between-group variation represents the variation (possibly systematic variation) between the treatment groups that is associated with the compound administered to each treatment group. The treatment groups were formed at randomization, and all of the subjects in one group receive the drug while all of the subjects in the other group receive the placebo. If the drug treatment group responses differ, on average, from the placebo treatment group responses, this suggests the possibility that the drug may be exerting an influence on SBP responses that is not exerted by the placebo.

Within-group variation represents the variation in SBP responses within each treatment group that is due to chance, i.e., random variation that is not caused by the compound administered to the treatment groups. This variation arises because humans have innate variation (as noted earlier, our biological systems operate such that we do not react identically in identical circumstances occurring at different times) and because all humans are different from each other. Within-group variation is not directly related to the treatment administered, since every subject in each group receives the same treatment.

6.4.4 Comparing Between-Group Variance and Within-Group Variance

Between-group variance can be called the effect variance, and within-group variance can be called the error variance. The effect variance is directly associated with the treatment administered, while the error variance is due to chance alone. The larger the effect variance when compared with the error variance, the more likely it is that compelling evidence of systematic variation will be revealed by inferential statistical analysis. Conversely, the smaller the effect variance when compared with the error variance, the less likely it is that compelling evidence of systematic variation will be revealed.

A useful way to compare any two quantities is to form a ratio by dividing one by the other. Since evaluation of the effect variance is the primary goal, this term is divided by the error variance:

Equation 6.1:

$$\text{Ratio of interest} = \frac{\text{effect variance (between-group variance)}}{\text{error variance (within-group variance)}}$$

There are three possibilities once this ratio has been calculated. If the effect variance is larger than the error variance, this ratio will produce a value that is larger than unity, i.e., larger than 1. If the effect variance turns out to be the same as the error variance (an extremely unlikely occurrence), the ratio will produce a value exactly equal to 1. And, if the effect variance is smaller than the error variance, this ratio will produce a value that is less than 1.

In statistical analyses, this ratio is called a test statistic. It is a numerical representation of the relative magnitudes of the effect variance and the error variance. In each circumstance in which a statistical analysis is applied, the test statistic has to reach a certain magnitude for the analysis to provide compelling evidence of systematic variation. The process for determining whether a test statistic has reached the necessary magnitude is discussed in detail in Chapter 7.

6.4.5 The Term "Error" Does Not Imply a "Mistake"

It is important to note here that the term "error" does not imply a mistake. It simply refers to the fact that, had a different random sample been taken from the same population, a different sample mean would have been obtained. Indeed, the words "error" and "random" are synonymous in many instances in Statistics. Error variance is variance due to random chance, as opposed to systematic variance that is the result of a systematic influence on the data. The term "randomization" as discussed in Chapter 5 describes a process whose purpose is to distribute error variance evenly across treatment groups so that it does not cloud our ability to detect any systematic variation that may be present.

6.5 PROBABILITY

In situations where certainty is not possible, it can be helpful to assess how likely it is that something will occur. Quantification of this likelihood is particularly helpful in statistical analysis. The concept of probability is used in everyday language, if rather more loosely than in Statistics. The statement "I'll probably be there on Saturday" involves a probabilistic statement, but there is no precise degree of quantification. If you know the individual making this statement, past experience may lead you to an informed judgment concerning the relative meaning of "probably," but this is a subjective judgment, not a quantitative statement.

In Statistics, a probability is a numerical quantity between zero and one that expresses the likely occurrence of a future event: Past events cannot be associated with a probability of occurrence, since it is known in absolute terms whether they occurred or not. A probability of zero denotes that the event will not (cannot) occur. A probability of one denotes that the event will undoubtedly occur. Any numerical value between zero and one expresses a relative likelihood of an event occurring. Additionally, the decimal expression of a probability value can be multiplied by 100 to create a percentage statement of likelihood. A probability of 0.5 would thus be expressed as a 50% chance that an event would occur. Similarly, and more relevantly for later discussions, probabilities of 0.05 and 0.01 would be expressed as a 5% chance and a 1% chance, respectively, that an event would occur.

6.5.1 Likely Events Don't Always Happen

While the probability of an event occurring can be specified precisely, the actual outcome is still a chance occurrence. Given that a coin has two sides, if a fair coin is tossed in the air, the chance that it will be a "heads" is one in two, or 0.5 (50%). However, there is no guarantee that a heads will result on any specified occasion. Therefore, while the probability value is our best numerical representation of the likelihood of a given outcome, in a specific case that outcome may not occur. A very high probability of, say, 0.95 for a given event does not actually guarantee the actual occurrence of that event, since 0.95 is less than 1.00. However, it is legitimate to interpret this probability as saying that we would expect it to occur 95 times out of a hundred opportunities to occur.

6.5.2 Clinical Decision Making

Clinical decision making also utilizes probability considerations, but these considerations can involve an extra degree of complexity in that they are often linked to the nature of a particular outcome as well as the probability of the outcome occurring. Consider a physician and patient deciding together whether a new drug would be a useful therapy for the patient. Imagine that clinical research during the drug's development indicates that a particular side effect is likely to occur in 5% of patients who take the drug. If this drug would be particularly useful in the management of the patient's condition, and the side effect is relatively benign (e.g., occasional moderate headaches), the clinician and the patient may decide that the risk of the side effect is worth taking. The side effect is relatively unlikely, and its occurrence would be manageable.

Consider now a similar scenario in which a different side effect also has a 5% probability of occurring but the side effect is extremely debilitating. The patient and the clinician may make a different decision this time. On balance, the potential benefit of the drug may not outweigh the risk of experiencing the relatively unlikely but very undesirable side effect. The issue of balancing benefit with risk is a common element of clinical practice, and the "benefit-to-risk ratio" represents an attempt to quantify this important balancing task. The benefits always need to outweigh the risks: Determining just how much the benefits need to outweigh the risks in a given situation is the province of clinical judgment and the clinician-patient relationship.

6.5.3 Sampling Theory

The goal of new drug development is to produce a marketed drug that will be beneficial to a very large number of individuals in a particular population, e.g., people with hypertension. (This statement is certainly true historically, and still true in many cases, but exciting new developments in the field of pharmacogenomics, as discussed in Chapter 20, mean that some new drug development may be targeted for an identifiable subgroup of a particular population.) Since around 50 million people in the United States have high blood pressure, it is simply not feasible to conduct a clinical trial of a new antihypertensive drug using all of these people. A sample of individuals is therefore chosen from the population of people with hypertension, and these subjects participate in the randomized clinical trial. While this trial provides precise numerical statements of the drug's effects in this specific sample, interest lies with the drug's likely effect in the population of hypertensives. In order for the results obtained from the subject sample (in the order of several thousand subjects) to generalize to the population with the disease condition of interest, the sample needs to represent the population as closely as possible.

6.5.4 The Standard Error of the Mean

In clinical research it is of particular interest to estimate a population mean on the basis of data collected from a sample of subjects employed in a randomized clinical trial. Sampling and statistical procedures facilitate the estimation of the population mean based on the sample mean and sample SD that are precisely calculated from the data collected in the trial. If we take a sample of 100 numbers from a population of 100,000 numbers and calculate the mean of those 100 numbers, this sample mean, which is precisely known, provides an estimate of the unknown population mean. If we then took another sample of 100 numbers, or indeed many samples, it is extremely unlikely that the numbers in any subsequent sample would be identical to those in the first sample, and it is unlikely that the calculated sample means would be identical to that of the first sample. Therefore, in a randomized clinical trial, a situation in which only one sample is taken from a population, a question that arises is: What degree of certainty is there that the mean of that sample represents the mean of the population? This question can be answered using statistical theory in conjunction with knowledge of the number of subjects participating in the trial, i.e., the sample size.

The larger the sample size, the more likely it is that the sample mean is a good representation of the population mean: If the sample were large enough to contain the entire population, the sample mean would be identical to the population mean. In a clinical trial, the sample size is precisely known. Knowledge of the sample SD and the sample size (*N*) facilitates precise calculation of the sample standard error of the mean (SEM):

Equation 6.2:
$$\text{SEM} = \frac{\text{SD}}{\sqrt{N}}$$

The SEM describes the degree of uncertainty present in the assessment of the population mean on the basis of the sample mean. This degree of uncertainty is due to sampling error. Conversely, it facilitates statements of the degree of certainty associated with the results obtained from a single sample.

With regard to the question of how well a single sample mean estimates the population mean, the question can be phrased as such: How different from the mean of the original sample would any other sample mean be? To answer this question, the mean of a sample is often presented along with its SEM, which (inversely) captures the degree of certainty in this estimation of the population mean. The smaller the SEM, the greater the degree of certainty with which the sample mean estimates the population mean. As can be seen from Equation 6.2, as *N* increases, the SEM of a given mean decreases. Therefore, the larger the sample size, the more likely it becomes that a given sample mean is a good estimate of the population mean.

6.6 THE NORMAL DISTRIBUTION

If the heights of a large number of adult males or adult females were measured and the results plotted as a histogram, the results would look something like Figure 6.1. This figure is presented for illustrative purposes only, and the lack of detailed information on the axes is not recommended for actual figures.

The key point to note in this figure is that there are many more people who are close to the middle of the histogram than there are people close to either end of the histogram. That is, more individuals are close to the mean height, and very few are very tall or very short. Given a large sample and decreasingly thin bars (that is, the width of the measurement intervals along the x-axis becomes infinitely small such that the height data become continuous), a curve can be superimposed on this histogram. This curve is called a density curve and is shown in Figure 6.2.

One particular version of a density curve is called the normal distribution. Height and many physiological variables conform closely (not perfectly) to this distribution. Since the word "normal" is used in everyday language, and since its meaning in Statistics is different and very important, the word "Normal" is written in this book with an upper case "N" when it is used in its statistical sense.

The Normal distribution has several notable properties:

- The highest point of the Normal curve occurs for the mean of the population. The properties of the Normal distribution ensure that this point is also the median value and the mode.

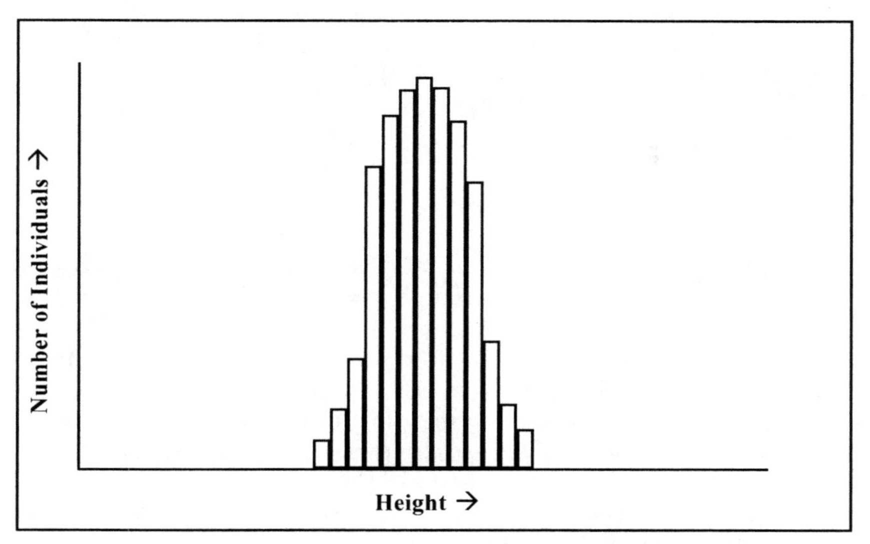

Figure 6.1. Heights of a random sample of adult males.

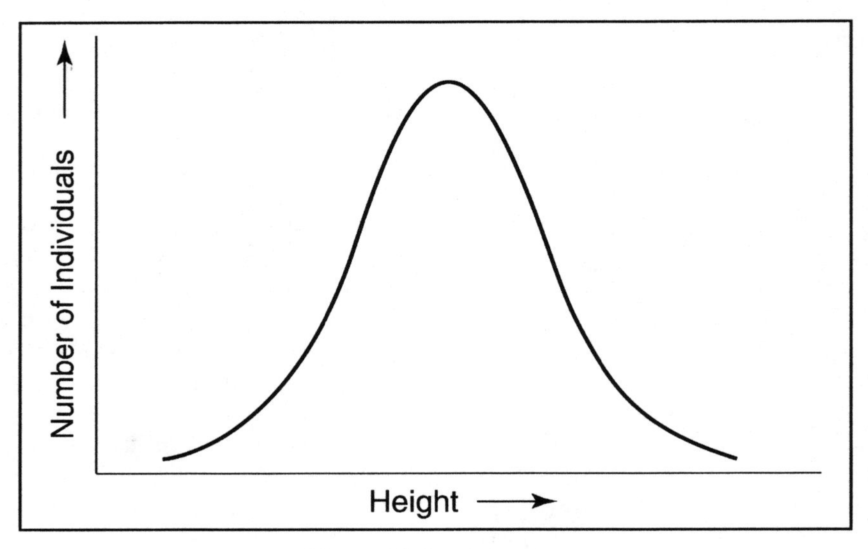

Figure 6.2. Density curve.

- The shape of the Normal curve (relatively narrow or relatively broad) is influenced by the SD of the data. The sides of the curve descend more gently as the SD increases and more steeply as it decreases.
- At a distance of approximately ±2 SDs from the mean, the slopes of the downward curves change from a relatively smooth downward slope to a curve that extends out to infinity and thus never quite reaches the x-axis. For practical purposes, the curve is often regarded as intercepting the x-axis at a distance of ±3 SDs from the mean, but this is an approximation.

This final point is expanded upon in Section 6.6.1.

6.6.1 Area Under the Normal Curve

The area under the Normal curve is of considerable interest in Statistics. That is, it is of considerable interest to define and quantify the area bounded by the Normal curve at the top and the x-axis at the bottom. This area will be defined as 1.0, or as 100%. Given this interest, the final point in Section 6.6 raised an issue that appears problematic. That is, it appears that, if the two lower slopes of the Normal curve never quite reach the x-axis, the area under the curve is never actually fully defined and can therefore never be calculated precisely. Fortunately, this apparent paradox can be solved mathematically. In the Preface of this book I noted that, in several cases, I had resisted the temptation to provide an explanation of subtle points. This case, I believe, is a worthwhile exception. An understanding of the qualities of the Normal distribution and the Normal curve is extremely helpful in setting the scene for topics covered in Chapters 7 and 8, namely statistical significance and clinical significance.

The solution is related to the observation that the sum of an infinite series can converge to a finite solution. An example that effectively demonstrates the solution here is the geometric series "1/2 + 1/4 + 1/8 + ... *ad infinitum*." That is, the series starts with 1/2, and every subsequent term is one half of the previous term. Given this, the terms of the series never vanish to zero. However, the sum of them is precisely 1. The proof of this is as follows, where the series is represented as S:

Equation 6.3: $S = 1/2 + 1/4 + 1/8 + \ldots$ *ad infinitum*

Both sides of this equation are then multiplied by the same value, namely 2 (multiplying both sides of an equation by a constant means that the sides are still of equal value):

Equation 6.4: $2S = 1 + 1/2 + 1/4 + \ldots$ *ad infinitum*

The value S is then subtracted from both sides (subtracting a constant from both sides of an equation means that the sides are still of equal value). First, consider the left hand side of Equation 6.4:

LHS of Equation 6.4: $2S - S$, which equals S

Now, consider the right hand side of Equation 6.4. Subtracting S from this quantity can be represented as

RHS of Equation 6.4: ($1 + 1/2 + 1/4 + \ldots$ *ad infinitum*) $- S$, which equals ?

To determine the value of "?," we can use Equation 6.3. That equation shows that S is equal to ($1/2 + 1/4 + 1/8 + \ldots$*ad infinitum*). Therefore, the right hand side of Equation 6.4 can be written as: "$(1 + S) - S$".

RHS of Equation 6.4: $(1 + S) - S$, which equals 1

Equation 6.4 can therefore be rewritten as:

$$S = 1$$

Therefore, despite the initial paradoxical nature of the statement, it can indeed be shown that the sum of an infinite series can converge to a finite solution.

Turning back to the focus of our interest here, the area under the Normal curve, the statement that the terms of the geometric series never vanish to zero can be reinterpreted in this context as saying that the curves of the Normal curve never intercept the x-axis. Despite this statement, an adaptation of the proof just provided shows that the area under the Normal curve is indeed precisely equal to 1, or 100%. The visual equivalent of this is that there is indeed a defined area under the Normal curve, bounded by the curve and the x-axis, and the value of this area can be represented as 1, or 100%.

6.6.2 Various Areas Under the Normal Curve

Of particular interest in Statistics is that the means of many large samples taken from a particular population are approximately distributed in this Normal fashion, i.e., they are said to be Normally distributed. This is true even when the population data themselves are not Normally distributed. The mathematical properties of a true Normal distribution allow quantitative statements of the area under the curve between any two points on the x-axis. In Section 6.6.1 it was shown that the total area under the Normal curve is 1, or 100%. It is also of interest to know the proportion of the total area under the curve that lies between two points that are equidistant from the mean. These points are typically represented by multiples of the SD. From the properties of the mathematical equation that governs the shape of the Normal curve, it can be shown that:

- 90% of the area under the curve lies between the mean ± 1.645 SDs
- 95% of the area under the curve lies between the mean ± 1.960 SDs
- 99% of the area under the curve lies between the mean ± 2.576 SDs

The area under the curve is representative of the number of data points falling within that range. That is, the percentage of the area under the curve translates directly into the percentage of data points falling between the two identified points. Of particular relevance for the discussions in subsequent chapters is that 95% of the area under the curve lies between the mean ±1.960 SDs. The value of 1.960 is often rounded up to 2.000, leading to the statement that 95% of the data points fall within ±2 SDs of the mean. The implications of this statement, and its fundamental importance in hypothesis testing and determination of clinical significance, will be picked up in Chapters 7 and 8.

6.7 Analysis of Association

It is often of interest to know if two variables are associated, and, if so, to what degree. In cases like this, the data set to be analyzed will consist of a certain number of pairs of data.

6.7.1 Nature (Direction) of an Association

Consider the example of age and weight in children. As a general statement, it would be fair to say that age and weight are associated. This statement alone, however, does not tell us how they are related or how closely they are related. A more informative general statement is that as age increases, weight increases. This statement provides information about the direction of the relationship between these two variables. An association where one variable increases as the other variable increases is called a positive association.

Consider now another example, the relationship between the age of a car and the car's monetary value. As a general statement, it is fair to say that a car's age and its value are associated. Again, this statement alone does not say how they are related or how closely they are related. A more informative general statement is that the value of a car decreases as the age of the car increases. An association where one variable decreases as the other variable increases is called a negative association.

6.7.2 Degree of Closeness of an Association

Consider first the example of a positive association. In the case of children's age and weight, these variables are not "perfectly" associated, since there are children of the same age who differ in weight. Consider now the example of a negative association. The age of a car and its value are also not "perfectly" related: Initially identical cars may have been maintained very differently, such that, when they are both five years old, one is worth much more than the other. The degree of closeness of an association is a separate characteristic of the relationship between two variables than is the direction of their association. There are close and less close positive associations and close and less close negative associations.

The degree of closeness between two variables can be described numerically via the statistical technique of correlation. The test statistic r is used in this statistical test and is known as the correlation coefficient. The correlation coefficient that is obtained from a correlational analysis reveals whether there is a statistically significant degree of association between the two variables. The magnitude of the correlation coefficient represents the degree of relationship between the variables. The larger the magnitude of the correlation coefficient, the more likely it is to attain statistical significance. A statistically significant result is interpreted as compelling evidence for the existence of a meaningful relationship between the variables.

6.7.3 Correlation Coefficients

Numerically, correlation coefficients can range from -1 to $+1$. A value of -1 indicates a "perfect" negative linear relationship; as one variable increases, the other decreases in a precise linear fashion. A value of 0 indicates a complete lack of linear association between two variables. A value of $+1$ indicates a "perfect" positive linear relationship; as one variable increases, the other increases in a precisely linear fashion. (The technique of correlation cannot meaningfully describe nonlinear patterns of association between two variables, such as curvilinear and exponential relationships.)

For continuous data, the Pearson product moment correlation coefficient, r, is calculated. Since continuous data are used here, certain fundamental assumptions are made, as for all parametric tests. It is assumed that both of the variables of interest are reasonably Normally distributed. The term "bivariate Normal" is used to describe data conforming to this assumption. This assumption can be checked visually by plotting a scattergram of all of the points in the sample. For a sample of data where both variables are distributed Normally, the imaginary outline drawn around all of these points is circular or elliptical (Fowler, Jarvis, and Chevannes, 2002). The more closely related the variables are, the more elliptical this outline becomes. Ultimately, in the case of a perfect linear association, the ellipse becomes a straight line.

6.7.4 Determining the Significance of a Product Moment Coefficient

Like all other test statistics discussed in this book, there is a probability distribution associated with the correlation coefficient, and, as usual, the degrees of freedom associated with the test statistic need to be determined in order to assess whether or not the test statistic attains statistical significance. In this case, the value for the degrees of freedom is N minus 2. This value is related to the fact that any two points lie on a straight line, and a third is needed to determine whether or not the points all lie on the same line. Degrees of freedom are discussed in Section 7.6.1.

The format of presenting a correlation coefficient is

$$r(18) = 0.80, p{=}0.02$$

In this case, there were 20 pairs of data, the correlation was 0.80, and the p-value attained statistical significance. As will be discussed in Chapter 7, a p-value of less than 0.05 indicates statistical significance. This result therefore represents compelling evidence that the two variables of interest are positively related. By convention, positive values typically are not preceded by a "+" sign: The absence of any sign is taken as a "+" sign. In contrast, if the correlation coefficient had been minus 0.80, the negative sign would be presented, and there would have been compelling evidence that the two variables of interest were negatively related.

6.7.5 The Coefficient of Determination

A measure called the coefficient of determination can be calculated as the proportion of the variability in one variable that is accounted for by variability in the other. The coefficient of determination is simply the square of the correlation coefficient. In the case of a perfect correlation, either positive (1.0) or negative (minus 1.0), the coefficient of determination will be identical to the correlation coefficient. This is also true for a correlation coefficient of zero. In any other case, the coefficient of determination will always be smaller than the correlation coefficient, since a value of less than 1 multiplied by itself results in a smaller value.

Thus, a correlation of 0.80 results in a coefficient of determination of 0.64. This value is typically expressed as 64%, and a statement is made that 64% of the variation in one variable, A, is accounted for by variance in the other variable, B. It therefore follows that 36% of the variance in A is not accounted for by variance in B and that at least one other factor is exerting an influence on the value of variable A.

Calculation of the coefficient of determination makes it very clear that a correlation coefficient of a certain magnitude does not represent an association that is "twice as strong" as an association represented by a correlation coefficient of half that magnitude. Consider the correlation coefficients 0.60 and 0.30. The coefficient of determination in the first case is 0.36, and, in the second case, the coefficient of determination is 0.09. The strength of association represented by a correlation coefficient of 0.60 is therefore considerably more than "twice the strength of association" represented by a correlation coefficient of 0.30. Note that the coefficient of determination for a correlation coefficient of 0.60 is exactly four times the coefficient of determination for a correlation of 0.30. This will be the case for any two correlation coefficients where one is exactly twice the size of the other. Since the correlation coefficient is squared to produce the coefficient of determination, the magnitude of the coefficient of determination for any correlation coefficient that is twice the magnitude of another will always be four times as great. Comparing correlations of determination is a more meaningful way of comparing strengths of association between sets of variables than is comparing correlation coefficients.

6.7.6 Association Does Not Necessarily Equate to Causation

While a large magnitude correlation coefficient calculated for two variables indicates a strong association between them, it does not make any statement about a causal relationship. That is, it does not imply a cause-and-effect relationship. There may indeed be such a relationship between the variables, but this cannot be determined from knowledge of the correlation coefficient alone. It is entirely possible that a third variable is systematically influencing both variables and is responsible for the strong correlation that is evident between them.

7

Statistical Significance: Employment of Hypothesis Testing

7.1 Introduction

As has been noted several times, one of the basic approaches in new drug development is to administer the test drug to one group of subjects, a placebo to another, and then see if the responses to the drug are, on average, different from those to the placebo. Providing a widely accepted answer to the question "Are the responses different?" requires framing the question in statistical language. Statistical techniques can then provide a quantitative determination of whether or not the responses are likely to be truly different. This is the realm of hypothesis testing, inferential statistics, and statistical significance.

7.2 Creating a Research Question and Associated Hypotheses

In Chapter 5, the importance of asking a useful research question was emphasized. A research question needs two qualities to be useful: it needs to be specific (precise) and to be testable. A general question such as "Is this drug good for people's blood pressure?" is not useful in this context. Using the continuing example of testing a new antihypertensive, the research question may be "Does the new drug alter SBP more than placebo?" Once this research question has been formulated, two hypotheses are created, the research hypothesis and the null hypothesis.

7.2.1 The Research Hypothesis

The research hypothesis typically reflects what is "hoped for," which in this case is that the drug undergoing testing will indeed alter SBP. In strict scientific terms, hope has no place in experimental research. The goal is to discover the truth, whatever it may be, and one should not start out hoping to find one particular outcome. In the real world, this ideologically pure stance is not common for many reasons (financial reasons being not the least of them). In this case, the research question is "Does the new drug alter SBP more than placebo?" The research hypothesis would be "The test drug alters SBP more than placebo."

7.2.2 The Null Hypothesis

The second hypothesis of interest here is called the null hypothesis. This is the counterpart of the research hypothesis. In this case, it states that "The test drug

New Drug Development: Design, Methodology, and Analysis. By J. Rick Turner

does not alter SBP more than placebo." The null hypothesis is actually the crux of hypothesis testing. For this reason, sometimes the null hypothesis is presented first, followed by the alternative hypothesis. The alternative hypothesis is simply another name for the research hypothesis, and therefore also states that "The test drug alters SBP more than placebo." The process of hypothesis testing can therefore be viewed as consisting of a null hypothesis accompanied by an alternative hypothesis, or as consisting of a research hypothesis accompanied by a null hypothesis. With no claim to authoritativeness, I prefer the latter, since the terms research question and research hypothesis fit together well. (This preference does not minimize the central role of the null hypothesis in hypothesis testing in any way.) Accordingly, subsequent discussions are structured such that the research question is presented first, followed by the research hypothesis, followed by the null hypothesis.

7.3 PRECISE EXPRESSION OF THE RESEARCH HYPOTHESIS AND THE NULL HYPOTHESIS: THE CONCEPT OF STATISTICAL SIGNIFICANCE

Imagine that, in a randomized clinical trial, the mean decrease in SBP for the drug treatment group was 4 mmHg and the mean decrease in SBP for the placebo treatment group was 3 mmHg (it is not unusual to see a relatively small mean decrease in blood pressure in a placebo treatment group). The research hypothesis as worded in Section 7.2 said "The test drug alters SBP more than placebo." Given these hypothetical data—mean decreases in SBP of 4 mmHg and 3 mmHg for the drug treatment group and the placebo treatment group, respectively—this hypothesis would appear to be true, since the mean decrease for the drug treatment group was 1 mmHg greater. The question here becomes: How much credence should be assigned to a difference of only 1 mmHg? Expressed differently, what level of confidence do we have that this is a "real" difference?

The issue here is one of deciding at what point an observed difference between treatment group means is sufficiently different that we believe a real difference exists, rather than believing that the difference is small enough that it could have occurred by chance alone.

You may think that this difference of 1 mmHg between the groups is so small that it is not real. The next question then becomes: Given that the placebo treatment group showed a mean decrease of 3 mmHg, what would the drug treatment group's mean decrease need to be for you to believe that it really was greater? 6 mmHg? 8 mmHg? 10 mmHg? Also, do you think that a colleague would agree with you? Statistical testing means that any subjectivity is removed, since the regulatory, scientific, and clinical communities accept the results obtained. That is, for a given set of data, statistical testing provides a precise statistical answer that has effectively been agreed upon as objective.

The concept of statistical significance facilitates this objectivity by expressing the outcome of a test in a way that everyone has agreed to honor. The words "significant," "significance," and "significantly" are used in everyday language in a meaningful but qualitative manner. In contrast, in Statistics they are used in a meaningful and quantitative manner. The appropriate statistical test will provide one of two answers. One possible answer says that the group means differ statistically significantly, allowing the statement to be made that this difference is unlikely to be the result of chance alone. The second possible answer says that the group means do not differ statistically significantly; this answer can be given even though the group means will almost certainly differ somewhat. This answer allows the statement to be made that this difference could well have arisen by chance alone.

The concept of statistical significance therefore allows the initial version of the research question, "Does the new drug alter SBP more than placebo?" to be reframed as follows: "Does the new drug alter SBP statistically significantly more than placebo?" It therefore facilitates the reframing of the research hypothesis and the null hypothesis in the same manner. The research hypothesis associated with the modified (improved) research question is framed as follows:

- The new drug alters SBP statistically significantly more than the placebo.

The null hypothesis associated with the improved research question is framed as follows:

- The new drug does not alter SBP statistically significantly more than the placebo.

Once the research hypothesis and the null hypothesis have been created, the process of hypothesis testing can take place.

7.4 HYPOTHESIS TESTING

As was noted in Section 7.2.2, the null hypothesis is the crux of hypothesis testing. Hypothesis testing revolves around two actions following an appropriate statistical analysis: rejecting the null hypothesis, or failing to reject the null hypothesis. The following sections explain the rationale behind the strategy of either rejecting the null hypothesis or failing to reject the null hypothesis. Statistical methodology necessitates a choice being made here: It is a forced choice paradigm. One of these two actions—rejecting the null hypothesis or failing to reject the null hypothesis —will occur at the end of all hypothesis testing. The action taken is determined by the statistical significance of the test statistic obtained in the statistical analysis.

7.5 CONDUCTING A STATISTICAL TEST AND OBTAINING A TEST STATISTIC

Statistical analyses result in a test statistic being calculated. For example, two common tests that will be introduced in this chapter are the *t*-test and a test called analysis of variance (ANOVA). The *t*-tests result in a test statistic called *t*, and ANOVA results in a test statistic called *F*. When you read the Results sections of regulatory submissions and clinical communications, you will become very familiar with these test statistics. The test statistic obtained determines whether the result of the statistical test attains statistical significance or not.

Consider our usual example, a parallel group design randomized clinical trial of a new drug, in which one group of subjects receives the drug for a specified period of time and the other group of subjects receives the placebo for an equal length of time. There are two statistical analyses that can be used here. One is the independent groups *t*-test, and the other is the one-factor independent groups ANOVA. Not surprisingly, since they are both appropriate, these two tests are intimately related and will yield precisely the same information. The values of the test statistics obtained from the respective tests will be different (the *F*-test statistic will be square of the *t*-test statistic), but the tests will give precisely the same answer in terms of the degree of statistical significance obtained by the respective test statistic, since the associated *p*-values will be identical. Therefore, both would lead to the same choice in terms of rejecting the null hypothesis or failing to reject the null hypothesis. In practical terms, the *t*-test, which can only be used when there are two treatment groups, is often chosen in this context. The advantage of the ANOVA approach becomes evident in situations where there are more than two treatment groups in a study, since ANOVA can handle this situation too. The ANOVA approach is discussed in Section 7.8.

7.6 THE INDEPENDENT GROUPS *t*-TEST

The independent groups *t*-test compares two sets of measurements that have been collected from two independent treatment groups, which is the case in the parallel group design employed in our ongoing example. The drug treatment group and the placebo treatment group were formed via randomization, and subjects in each group received only one or the other treatment. The two groups of subjects are therefore independent, hence the connection with the name of this *t*-test. A corollary of this observation is that the independent groups *t*-test can be used when the numbers of subjects in the two treatment groups are different: The number of subjects in each treatment group is taken into account in the calculations involved in this test.

The major steps in the calculation and interpretation of this test are summarized as follows:

1. Calculate the mean change score for each treatment group.
2. Calculate the difference between the mean change score for the drug treatment group and the mean change score for the placebo group, i.e., the effect size.
3. Calculate the error variance.
4. Divide the effect size by the error variance to give the test statistic t.
5. Calculate the degrees of freedom associated with the t-value.
6. Determine the p-level associated with the t-value and its associated degrees of freedom.
7. Based on the p-level, reject the null hypothesis or fail to reject the null hypothesis.
8. Interpret the result in words in the context of the specific research question.

Before continuing, the concept of degrees of freedom, mentioned in point 5, is addressed.

7.6.1 Degrees of Freedom

Consider the following instruction: "Select any five numbers that add up to 100." How much choice is there in this selection? Only four numbers can be chosen freely. Once these have been chosen, the fifth number is determined by the four already chosen: Whatever the sum of the first four numbers, addition of the fifth must produce the number 100. That is, there are four "degrees of freedom" to your choice; four choices have freedom, the fifth does not.

Now consider the following instruction "Select any five numbers that have a mean of 20." While worded differently, this is an equivalent instruction since any five numbers that add up to 100 will have a mean of 20. Again, therefore, only four numbers can be chosen freely. Generalizing this concept in the context of present discussions, in a particular treatment group of size N with a given mean, there are N minus 1 degrees of freedom. In any study, the number of subjects in a given treatment group is known, and the mean of the measurement of interest (in this case the mean SBP change score) is known. In the present context, the degrees of freedom associated with the group's mean SBP change score are N minus 1.

Extending this to the ongoing example, there are two treatment groups of interest, and the number of subjects in each group is known (recall that these numbers can be different in the parallel group design). Let us refer to the number of subjects in these groups as N(treatment) and N(placebo). In each case, the number of degrees of freedom is N minus 1. The total number of degrees of freedom in the independent groups t-test is calculated as the sum of the degrees of freedom for each treatment group:

[*N*(treatment)-1] + [*N*(placebo)-1]

This can be expressed more succinctly as:

N(treatment) + *N*(placebo) -2

In Section 7.5, it was noted that the test statistic obtained at the end of a statistical analysis determines whether the result of the statistical test achieves statistical significance or not. This is a correct statement, but an incomplete one. The complete statement is that the test statistic obtained, in conjunction with the associated degrees of freedom, determines whether the result of the statistical test achieves statistical significance or not. It is quite possible that precisely the same test statistic will attain statistical significance in conjunction with one set of degrees of freedom and not attain statistical significance with another. The degrees of freedom associated with a given test statistic are not often cited in regulatory documents or in clinical communications, and so you may not see these very often in your own reading. Nonetheless, it is important to be aware that the level of statistical significance attained by a given test statistic is governed by the degrees of freedom associated with the test statistic. Therefore, the degrees of freedom are included in the examples provided here.

7.6.2 Format of Results from an Independent Groups *t*-Test

As an example, consider two groups of 10 subjects and 11 subjects, respectively. These group totals are clearly unrealistically small in terms of a randomized clinical trial, but they allow the methodology of the *t*-test to be demonstrated. Imagine that these hypothetical data represent SBP change scores:

- Drug treatment group SBP change scores (all decreases): 3, 0, 3, 8, 5, 9, 4, 7, 5, 6.
- Placebo treatment group SBP change scores (all decreases) : 4, 2, 2, 0, 1, 0, 1, 4, 3, 2, 3.

The steps involved in the calculation of the *t*-test were provided in Section 7.6. Following these steps:

1. The drug treatment group mean change score is 5.00 mmHg, and the placebo treatment group mean change score is 2.00 mmHg.
2. The difference between the treatment group means (the effect size) is 3.00 mmHg.
3. The error variance (calculated according to a formula that need not be presented here) is 0.9187.
4. The effect size divided by the error variance gives a test statistic of $t = 3.27$.

5. The degrees of freedom are *N*(Treatment) + *N*(Placebo) -2 = 10 + 11 – 2 = 19.

This result is written as $t(19) = 3.27$.

Completion of Step 6, "Determine the *p*-level associated with the *t*-value and its associated degrees of freedom," requires a little more groundwork. As noted earlier in this chapter, all statistical tests culminate in the calculation of a test statistic. However, this numerical value is not the final numerical answer from the statistical test. Another component of the numerical answer, the probability level associated with this numerical value, must be determined. Then, once the full numerical answer is obtained, the numerical answer must be interpreted, in words, in the context of the study. Before the advent of the personal computer, it was common to use a table of critical values to find this probability level. To attain a given level of statistical significance, typically $p<0.05$, the test statistic must be of a certain magnitude or greater. The respective table therefore documents what magnitude the test statistic must reach to be statistically significant at the $p<0.05$ level. (These tables usually include the $p<0.01$ level too and sometimes the $p<0.001$ level.) Use of these tables therefore established whether a given statistic was statistically significant at the $p<0.05$ level or not. These tables are still used for teaching purposes in Statistics courses, but, in real-life situations, the use of computers facilitates computation of the actual *p*-level associated with a given test statistic.

This approach yields additional information over and above that gained from tables of critical values, in that two test statistics that are both significant at the $p<0.05$ level may have associated probabilities that are quite different, e.g., $p=0.044$ and $p=0.012$. While both *p*-values are less than 0.05, the former is not that much less, while the latter is considerably less. This is why modern journal publishing practices prefer authors to provide the actual *p*-value associated with a test statistic.

7.6.3 The *p*-Value: Its Definition and Meaning

In the present example, an effect size of 3.00 mmHg was observed. That is, the difference between the drug treatment group mean change score and the placebo treatment group mean change score was 3.00 mmHg. This effect size has been precisely calculated on the basis of the data obtained in the clinical trial. Recall, however, that in a randomized clinical trial the subjects used are a random sample of all the people in the disease population of interest. Our interest actually lies with the effect size in that population. The population effect size is not known, and a question of interest is: How well does the effect size calculated in our sample reflect the unknown effect size in the population? This question is at the heart of inferential statistics.

The premise of inferential statistics is that, if data are carefully collected in a study that employs the appropriate design and methodology, analysis of these data allows us to infer what the population effect size is likely to be based on the effect size calculated for the subject sample that participated in the trial. The p-value that occurs at the end of this hypothesis testing strategy is the probability of finding an effect size of that magnitude, or greater, if the null hypothesis were true. The p-values are a central component of hypothesis testing.

The widely accepted cut-off for statistical significance is $p<0.05$. A p-value that is less than 0.05 means that, if the null hypothesis were true, the chance of finding an effect size of the magnitude seen or greater would be less than 5%. A result is typically declared statistically significant if the p-value associated with the test statistic is less than 0.05. There are other significance levels that are used, such as the $p<0.01$ level of significance. This is a more conservative level of significance, since it is harder to attain. A p-value of less than 0.01 means that, if the null hypothesis were true, the chance of finding an effect size of that magnitude or greater is less than 1%.

7.6.4 The p-Value and Hypothesis Testing

In Section 7.6, the steps involved in the calculation of the independent groups t-test were listed. The final three were:

6. Determine the p-level associated with the t-value and its associated degrees of freedom.
7. Based on the p-level, reject the null hypothesis or fail to reject the null hypothesis.
8. Interpret the result in words in the context of the specific research question.

Addressing step 6, the t-value that is given by this example is

$$t(19) = 3.27$$

Performing this test by computer would give the p-value associated with this value. The p-value is 0.004, and the full numerical result of the test is therefore written as

$$t(19) = 3.27, p=0.004$$

This p-value is less than 0.05 (and also less than 0.01, a more conservative significance level).

Step 7 states "Based on the p-level, reject the null hypothesis or fail to reject the null hypothesis." As discussed in Section 7.4, one of two actions—rejecting the null hypothesis or failing to reject the null hypothesis—occurs at the end of all hypothesis testing, and the action taken is determined by the statistical significance of the test statistic obtained in the statistical analysis. When statistical significance is attained, the null hypothesis is rejected in favor of the research hypothesis. The research hypothesis states that:

- The new drug alters SBP statistically significantly more than the placebo.

Step 8 states "Interpret the result in words in the context of the specific research question." Interpreting this result in the context of the specific aim of this study, it provides compelling evidence that the new drug alters SBP more than the placebo treatment.

7.6.5 Two More Examples of Results from an Independent Groups *t*-Test

Imagine that a randomized clinical trial was conducted to compare the mean change in SBP in the drug treatment group with the mean SBP change in the placebo treatment group, and the results were as follows:

- Mean SBP decrease for the drug treatment group = 8.1 mmHg.
- Mean SBP decrease for the placebo treatment group = 1.9 mmHg.
- Effect size (difference between the treatment group means) = 6.2 mmHg.
- p=0.020.

What is the message conveyed by these results? The p-value that occurs at the end of hypothesis testing is the probability of finding a difference of that size or greater between the drug treatment group mean change score and the placebo treatment group mean change score if the null hypothesis were true. The accepted cut-off for statistical significance is $p<0.05$. The p-value of 0.020 tells us that if the null hypothesis were true, the chance of getting a group difference of 6.2 mmHg is 2%. That is, if the null hypothesis were true, there is only a 2% chance (less than a 5% chance) of obtaining this result. Based on the unlikely occurrence of this result, the null hypothesis is rejected, and a statement made that, based on the subject sample used in this study, there is statistically compelling evidence that the drug would alter SBP in the general population of hypertensives.

Imagine now that the result from the same randomized clinical trial had been as follows:

- Mean SBP decrease for the drug treatment group = 2.7 mmHg.
- Mean SBP decrease for the placebo treatment group = 1.9 mmHg.
- Effect size (difference between the treatment group means) = 0.8 mmHg.
- p=0.640.

What is the statistical message conveyed by this result? If the null hypothesis were true, the chance of getting a group difference of 0.8 mmHg or greater is 64%. If the null hypothesis were true, there is greater than a 5% chance that we would get this result. The evidence is therefore not strong enough to reject the null hypothesis: that is, we fail to reject it. Accordingly, a statement is made that, based on the subject sample used in this clinical trial, there is no statistically compelling evidence that the drug would alter SBP in the general population of hypertensives.

7.7 THE DEPENDENT MEASURES *t*-TEST

There are two forms of the *t*-test, and each is applicable for sets of measurements that have been obtained in different ways. The method of data collection precisely and uniquely determines which of these two forms of statistical analysis is appropriate. Section 7.6 introduced the independent groups *t*-test, which is appropriate for the analysis of data collected during a study employing a parallel group study design. Another form of the *t*-test is called the dependent measures *t*-test. This test is sometimes called the related measures *t*-test, the repeated measures *t*-test, or the *t*-test for matched pairs. The name dependent measures *t*-test has been chosen here since the contrast with the word independent in the name "independent groups *t*-test" is clear.

The dependent measures *t*-test is appropriate for the analysis of data collected during a study employing a cross-over study design. This *t*-test compares two sets of measurements that are related in a special way. Each subject is administered both treatments and therefore provides data for each treatment group. Therefore, every measurement in one treatment group has a precise counterpart in the other treatment group. Imagine that subjects take part in a simple cross-over trial. Half of the subjects receive the drug treatment first, and half of them receive the placebo treatment first. Each subject therefore provides a measurement for both the drug treatment and the placebo treatment and therefore provides a pair of measurements that are related to each other in that they both came from the same subject. Using the nomenclature of this test, these pairs of measurements are dependent on each other in that they both came from the same subject.

The fact that data that are analyzed by this form of the *t*-test can be meaningfully paired dictates that there will always be the same number of measurements in each group. This inherent consistency contrasts with the independent groups *t*-test, where the two groups may or may not have the same numbers of measurements. Having made this observation, however, it is of critical importance to emphasize that the mere fact that two groups being compared contain the same number of measurements does not guarantee that the dependent measures *t*-test is the appropriate form of the *t*-test to use. The dependent measures *t*-test is only appropriate when the data in groups being compared can be meaningfully paired.

The dependent measures *t*-test uses the relationship between each pair of data in the steps necessary to calculate the test statistic t. Conceptually, the calculation of the test statistic is the same as for the independent groups *t*-test, as listed in Section 7.6:

1. Calculate the mean change score for each treatment group.
2. Calculate the difference between the mean change score for the drug treatment group and the mean change score for the placebo group, i.e., the effect size.
3. Calculate the error variance.
4. Divide the effect size by the error variance to give the test statistic t.
5. Calculate the degrees of freedom associated with the t-value.
6. Determine the p-level associated with the t-value and its associated degrees of freedom.
7. Based on the p-level, reject the null hypothesis or fail to reject the null hypothesis.
8. Interpret the result in words in the context of the specific research question.

In this case, some of the computational steps are different, since there is a relationship between pairs of data that does not exist in cases where the use of the independent groups t-test is appropriate. The computation of the error variance is performed in a different manner, and the value of the degrees of freedom associated with the test statistic is computed differently. Nevertheless, the basic objective, rejecting the null hypothesis or failing to reject the null hypothesis, is identical.

7.8 ANALYSIS OF VARIANCE

As noted in Section 7.5, one-factor independent groups ANOVA can also be used in cases where the independent groups t-test is appropriate. The term "independent groups" is derived in exactly the same way as was independent groups t-test, in that independent groups of subjects are employed. The term "one-factor" relates to the fact that, in our ongoing example, there is only one factor that is of interest: that factor is "type of treatment administered." A factor is an influence that one wishes to study; it is of interest to know whether the factor is a systematic source of influence on, and therefore a systematic source of variance in, the data collected in a study. An equivalent designation is not necessary in the case of the t-test, since it can only be used when there is just one factor of interest.

In contrast, the added sophistication of ANOVA does allow more than one factor to be studied at the same time. Imagine a scenario (not a particularly likely one, but the point can still be made) where it is of interest to study whether a drug is more effective when given in the morning than when given in the evening. In this case, two factors are of interest: type of treatment administered and time of day. In this scenario, each factor has two levels: drug treatment and placebo treatment and morning and evening, respectively. Therefore, there would be four independent groups of subjects in such a study: subjects receiving the drug treatment in the morning, the drug treatment in the evening, the placebo treatment in the morning, and the placebo treatment in the evening. Various other ANOVAs are appropriate for many other study designs, including quite complex designs that are relatively uncommon in clinical trials. Such designs, however, are commonly used in other fields of research, and the sophistication and flexibility inherent in ANOVA make it one of the most powerful and widely used statistical techniques in those fields. In this book, we will focus on relatively simple but very informative study designs in clinical trials for which ANOVA is very useful.

7.9 ONE-FACTOR INDEPENDENT GROUPS ANOVA

Consider a study where three doses of a new antihypertensive drug are to be compared, and three groups of subjects will each receive one dose. Such a study may be performed in earlier phase drug development to determine the most appropriate dose for subsequent larger trials. The research question, research hypothesis, and null hypothesis in this case would be:

- Research question: Does the dose of drug administered statistically significantly influence the change in SBP seen for the different doses?
- Research hypothesis: The dose of drug administered statistically significantly influences the change in SBP seen for the different doses.
- Null hypothesis: The dose of drug administered does not statistically significantly influence the change in SBP seen for the different doses

The simple fact that there are three treatment groups means that an independent groups *t*-test cannot be employed; that test can only handle two treatment groups. In this case, a one-factor independent groups ANOVA is appropriate. From now on, the "one-factor" part of the name will be left off, since our examples focus on designs where only one source of influence is being investigated.

7.9.1 The Test Statistic in ANOVA

As noted in Section 7.5, the test statistic in ANOVAs is called *F*, and the test is sometimes called the *F*-test. The name pays respect to Sir Ronald Fisher, the statistician who developed this approach. Similarly to the calculation of the test statistic *t* in a *t*-test, *F* is calculated as a ratio, as follows:

$$F = \frac{\text{effect variance}}{\text{error variance}} = \frac{\text{between treatment groups variance}}{\text{within treatment groups variance}}$$

Analogously to *t*, *F* has to reach a certain size to attain statistical significance. This size is dictated by the associated degrees of freedom in each instance, and in turn the degrees of freedom are dictated by the total number of subjects participating in the study. To attain significance, *F* must always be greater than 1, which means that the between-subjects variance (the effect variance) must be greater than the within-subject variance (the error variance).

7.9.2 Calculation of the *F*-Test

The major steps in the calculation and interpretation of the *F*-test are:

1. Calculate the mean change score for each of the treatment groups.
2. Calculate the between-groups variance.
3. Calculate the within-groups variance.
4. Divide the between-groups variance by the within-groups variance to give the test statistic *F*.
5. Calculate the degrees of freedom associated with the *F*-value.
6. Determine the *p*-level associated with the *F*-value and its associated degrees of freedom.
7. Based on the *p*-level, reject the null hypothesis or fail to reject the null hypothesis.
8. Interpret the result in words in the context of the specific research question.

In ANOVA, the test statistic *F* will have two associated degrees of freedom. One of these is associated with the between-groups variance and is determined by the number of treatment groups. This value will be 1 less than the total number of groups. The second value is associated with the within-groups variance. This value is the sum of the degrees of freedom associated with each of the treatment groups. For each treatment group, the degrees of freedom are 1 less than the number of subjects in that group.

To illustrate this process, imagine a study in which three groups of subjects receive one dose of an antihypertensive drug each, 10 mg, 20 mg, or 30 mg, and there are 20 subjects in each. The mean decreases in SBP for the three dose treatment groups are as follows:

- 10-mg dose treatment group: 3 mmHg
- 20-mg dose treatment group: 11 mmHg
- 30-mg dose treatment group: 12 mmHg

Imagine that the calculated *F*-value is 4.0. The degrees of freedom associated with this *F*-value come from the degrees of freedom associated with the between-groups variance and the within-groups variance. The degrees of freedom associated with the between-groups variance are (3 minus 1), i.e., 2. The degrees of freedom associated with the within-groups variance are (20 minus 1) + (20 minus 1) + (20 minus 1), i.e., 57. In this example, therefore, the *F*-value would be represented as:

$$F(2, 57) = 4.0$$

There will be a *p*-value associated with this *F*-value. Imagine that this *p*-value is 0.03. The final numerical result from the ANOVA would therefore be written as:

$$F(2, 57) = 4.0, p=0.03$$

As always, this numerical result must be interpreted in the context of this specific study. In this case, since there is a statistically significant result (the *p*-value is less than 0.05), the null hypothesis is rejected, and it is concluded that the dose of drug administered does statistically significantly influence the change in SBP.

However, this statement in itself does not tell us anything about the mean decreases in SBP for the three drug dose treatment groups. To address this, the mean decreases in SBP for the three groups, provided earlier in this Section, need to be considered. These were:

- 10-mg dose treatment group: 3 mmHg
- 20-mg dose treatment group: 11 mmHg
- 30-mg dose treatment group: 12 mmHg

Thus, the mean decrease for the 10-mg dose treatment group was the least, the mean decrease for the 20-mg dose treatment group was numerically greater, and the mean decrease for the 30-mg dose treatment group was numerically greater than both of the other two dose treatment groups.

Again, even this information does not provide the most comprehensive answer possible in this situation. In this context of more than two treatment groups, the ANOVA is called an omnibus test. It is an overall test of statistical significance. The statistically significant result says that, somewhere, there is at least one statistically significant difference between pairs of the dose treatment groups. There are three pairs of dose treatment groups to consider:

- The 10-mg dose treatment group and the 20-mg dose treatment group
- The 10-mg dose treatment group and the 30-mg dose treatment group
- The 20-mg dose treatment group and the 30-mg dose treatment group

The significant omnibus test does not reveal which of several possible patterns of statistically significant differences has occurred. Simple visual inspection may suggest that the 10-mg dose treatment group mean (a decrease in SBP of 3 mmHg) and the 20-mg dose treatment group mean (a decrease of 11 mmHg) may be meaningfully different and the 10-mg dose treatment group mean (a decrease of 3 mmHg) and the 30-mg dose treatment group mean (a decrease of 12 mmHg) may also be meaningfully different. The same visual inspection may also suggest that the 20-mg dose treatment group mean (a decrease of 11 mmHg) and the 30-mg dose treatment group mean (a decrease of 12 mmHg) may not be meaningfully different.

Given the carefully chosen mean changes used in this example, such a visual inspection may lead fairly readily to the suggestions above. However, in reality, the pattern of dose treatment group patterns is likely to be less sharply defined. Additionally, whether the pattern of dose response across treatment groups is relatively clear or not in a visual inspection, such inspection does not provide a statistical answer to the question of interest, i.e., which dose treatment group(s) differ significantly from which other dose treatment group(s). The answer to this question requires a further statistical analysis.

7.9.3 A Further Analytical Step: Multiple Comparisons

The significant F-value in Section 7.9.2 revealed that there is at least one statistically significant difference between a pair of dose treatment groups. However, given that there are more than two groups, it cannot reveal the precise pattern of statistical significance. This contrasts with the scenario where there are only two groups. If a significant F-value is obtained in an ANOVA when there are only two levels, there is only one possible interpretation: The two levels differ significantly from each other, and the group means reveal the direction of this difference. (This logic is precisely the same logic seen in t-tests.)

In situations such as the one introduced in Section 7.9.2, i.e., one in which an omnibus test reveals a partial answer to the research question, multiple comparisons are performed. These are tests that facilitate the comparison of the means of each pair of treatment groups to see which pair(s) differ statistically significantly from each other. Multiple comparisons therefore provide a more detailed understanding of data than is provided by the initial omnibus test. (In cases where an omnibus test yields a nonsignificant result, it is not appropriate to continue to perform multiple comparisons.)

There are various multiple-comparison strategies in the discipline of Statistics. One that is appropriate and illustrative in this case is the Tukey test. The first step in the Tukey test is to construct a trellis for the comparison of all sample means (Fowler et al., 2002). For each pair of comparisons, the mean of one dose treatment group is subtracted from the mean of the other. The sign (positive or negative) of the individual means must be taken into account in these calculations, but if the sign of the resulting difference is a negative sign, this can be ignored. Therefore, either mean can be subtracted from the other, since the resultant absolute value will be identical in both scenarios. Since the mean SBP changes for all three dose treatment groups in the example are actually decreases in SBP, negative signs are used in Table 7.1. For the comparison of the 10-mg group and the 20-mg group, the necessary calculation is

$$(-3) - (-11) = -3 + 11 = 8.$$

The other two calculations are performed similarly, and the resulting differences placed into the trellis shown in Table 7.1.

Table 7.1. Trellis for the Tukey Multiple Comparison Test

Dose Treatment Group & Group Mean	20 mg (-11 mmHg)	30 mg (-12 mmHg)
10 mg (-3 mmHg)	8	9
20 mg (-11 mmHg)	N/A	1

Next, the test statistic for this test is calculated. This test statistic is represented by the capital letter *T*. This test statistic is then used as a reference standard against which to compare each of the three differences between the means of pairs of groups presented in Table 7.1. Imagine that the value of *T* is calculated as 1.70. In this test, any value that is greater than the test statistic *T* is defined as being statistically significant at the 5% level. The results are therefore:

- 10-mg dose treatment group versus 20-mg dose treatment group = 8; $p<0.05$
- 10-mg dose treatment group versus 30-mg dose treatment group = 9; $p<0.05$
- 20-mg dose treatment group versus 30-mg dose treatment group = 1.

These results now provide the full numerical answer to the original research question. As always, the numerical results need to be interpreted in words in the context of the specific study. This interpretation requires combining the information from the Tukey test with the group means calculated earlier (10-mg dose treatment group = -3 mmHg; 20-mg dose treatment group = -11 mmHg; 30-mg dose treatment group = -12 mmHg).

The full interpretation of the results is:

- There is evidence at the 5% level that the mean SBP decrease for the 20-mg dose treatment group is significantly greater than the mean decrease for the 10-mg dose treatment group.
- There is evidence at the 5% level that the mean SBP decrease for the 30-mg dose treatment group is significantly greater than the mean decrease for the 10-mg dose treatment group.
- There is no statistical evidence that the mean SBP decrease for the 30-mg dose treatment group is significantly greater than the mean decrease for the 20-mg dose treatment group. (Note that this statement is made even though the mean SBP decrease for the 30-mg dose treatment group was actually numerically greater than that for the 20-mg dose treatment group.)

7.10 GENERAL COMMENTS ON MULTIPLE-COMPARISON TESTING

At this point, is it appropriate to address a reasonable question that you may be asking. Since each comparison in the Tukey test involves only two groups, and since we have already encountered a test that compares two groups perfectly adequately (the *t*-test), why not simply conduct three *t*-tests, one for each pair of groups that need to be compared?

The answer to this question concerns a potential problem when conducting multiple comparisons. As long as the appropriate statistical care is taken, the problem can be dealt with completely satisfactorily. However, simply performing three *t*-tests would not fulfill this criterion of taking appropriate statistical care. The potential problem is this: The more comparisons that are made, the more likely it becomes that a statistically significant result will erroneously be "found" by chance alone. When adopting the 5% significance level, it is likely that, if 20 separate comparisons are made, a statistically significant result will erroneously be "found" by chance alone. This statement is a direct result of the way that statistical hypothesis testing is structured.

In more general terms, the more tests that are performed, the more likely it becomes that one of them will erroneously be found to be significant. Therefore, it is not appropriate statistical practice to conduct many tests, find one statistically significant result, and present this lone result as a noteworthy finding. It is particularly not appropriate to present this result in the spirit that this is something that you anticipated all along (i.e., that this was identified *a priori* as a comparison of interest). If a situation occurs in which one of many tests is significant, and you believe that the result is biologically plausible and worthy of further investigation, a subsequent trial needs to be conducted, and this comparison needs to be genuinely identified *a priori* as the comparison of interest.

7.10.1 Type I Errors and Type II Errors

A Type I error is said to occur when a significant result is found when it does not really exist. Therefore, as noted, when conducting about 20 separate comparisons, it is likely that a Type I error will occur (i.e., a statistically significant result will erroneously be found by chance alone). A strategy has therefore been developed to counter this likelihood. This strategy involves using a more conservative approach to significance testing when multiple comparisons are made. A corollary of this strategy, however, is that it increases the likely occurrence of a Type II error, i.e., failing to find a significant difference that actually exists. The increased likelihood of a Type II error arises here because Type I and Type II errors are related in an inverse manner. All statistical testing has to balance the relative acceptability of Type I errors versus Type II errors. In the case of multiple-comparison testing, which involves testing multiple hypotheses via the calculation of multiple test statistics, a more conservative approach is deemed preferable.

The Tukey test is structured to take a conservative approach in an ingenious manner. Keeping all other considerations and variables constant, as the number of treatment groups increases (that is, as the number of comparisons being made increases), the size of the test statistic T increases. Since the difference between any two groups' means has to exceed the value of T for that test to attain statistical significance, the total number of comparisons being made determines the likelihood of that difference between the two groups' means attaining statistical significance. For a difference score of a given magnitude, the more comparisons that are made, the less likely it is that the difference will attain statistical significance.

7.11 POSSIBLE CLINICAL INTERPRETATIONS OF STATISTICAL RESULTS

The interpretations given in Section 7.9.3 are the full statistical interpretations from the analyses performed in this hypothetical study. In real clinical trials, an additional step in the interpretation of the trial's results would occur: The clinical significance of such results would be considered. Making clinical interpretations is the province of the clinicians on the study team. (I emphasize here that I am not a clinician, and my comments concerning any possible clinical significance, even for these hypothetical results, should be regarded in this light.) First, the clinical significance of the mean decreases in SBP seen in the three dose treatment groups must be considered. That is, is a decrease of 3 mmHg clinically significant, and are decreases of 12 mmHg and 13 mmHg clinically significant?

Suppose for the sake of this example that a decrease of 3 mmHg (while desirable, since all decreases are beneficial) was not considered clinically significant by the clinicians on the research team, while decreases of 11 mmHg and 12 mmHg were considered clinically significant. The hypothetical statistical results for this scenario revealed no statistical difference in the group means for the 20-mg dose treatment group and the 30-mg dose treatment group. That is, the 20-mg dose produced a mean decrease in SBP that was not statistically significantly different from the decrease produced by the 30-mg dose. Suppose that the safety data collected in this trial had shown that the 30-mg dose led to considerable more AEs than the 20-mg dose. Combining statistical interpretations and clinical judgments with inspection of the safety data, it might be argued that the 20-mg dose of this particular antihypertensive drug is preferable to the 30-mg dose. The rationale for this argument would be that the 20-mg dose produces a decrease in SBP that is not statistically significantly different from the decrease produced by the 30-mg dose, and it is safer.

In real life, clinical interpretations need to balance the relative weights of safety and efficacy considerations. If a higher dose of a given drug is considerably more effective than a lower dose and it only leads to a minimal increase in very mild side effects, a clinician may decide that, on balance, it is worth recommending the higher dose. Conversely, if a higher dose of a given drug is only minimally more effective than a lower dose and it leads to a considerable increase in moderate or severe side effects, a clinician may recommend the lower dose. (A similar issue was addressed in Section 6.5.2.) The scientific discipline of Statistics can provide clear evidence of the presence or absence of statistical significance between treatment options for clinicians to consider, but clinical practice also requires careful consideration and evaluations of this evidence and then making decisions that can be much less clear-cut. For this reason, clinical practice can meaningfully be regarded as an art as well as a science: Along with optimum quality data, experience and well-developed decision-making skills are invaluable. This topic is discussed further in Chapter 13.

8

Clinical Significance: Employment of Confidence Intervals

8.1 Introduction

While hypothesis testing is very informative, and is sufficient in some circumstances, it is not sufficient in the clinical arena. Gardner and Altman (1986) commented that "presenting *p*-values alone can lead to them being given more merit than they deserve. In particular, there is a tendency to equate statistical significance with medical importance or biological relevance." Statistical significance must not be equated with medical importance or biological relevance. In the clinical arena, the use of confidence intervals (CIs) is very meaningful, and their presentation is an important component of regulatory documentation and clinical communications. Confidence intervals facilitate quantification of the degree of confidence that is placed in the estimation of a treatment effect. The properties of the Normal distribution (discussed in Section 6.6) allow statements concerning the value of the population treatment effect to be made with specified degrees of certainty based on the data collected in a single clinical trial.

8.2 The Logic of Confidence Intervals

When a randomized clinical trial is conducted, a subject sample is chosen from the population of all possible subjects, and this sample is then randomized to the treatment groups. Analysis of the trial's data provides a precise result for that particular sample. However, importantly, while the sample can contain several thousand subjects, this is quite likely to be a very small percentage of the population from which that sample was chosen. Had a different sample of subjects been chosen, the chances of the data obtained being identical is so infinitesimally small that we can safely say that they would be different. The question of interest here is: How different would they likely be? Ideally, we would like them to be extremely similar, thus providing a result that is extremely similar to the result of the original trial; the more similar the results from a second trial, the more confidence we could reasonably place in the results from the original trial.

While the word "confidence" in the previous sentence occurs in its everyday use, the term is also used in Statistics in a precise manner, analogously to the statistical terms "Normal" and "significant." Confidence intervals constitute a range of values that are defined by the lower limit and the upper limit of the interval. These limits are symmetrically placed on either side of the sample mean. A commonly used CI is the 95% CI. A commonly expressed view of a 95% CI is that one can be 95% certain that

New Drug Development: Design, Methodology, and Analysis. By J. Rick Turner

the range defined by the lower and upper limits of this interval contains the "true" mean for the entire population. A more precise definition is provided in Section 8.3.1.

8.3 CONFIDENCE INTERVALS FOR A SAMPLE MEAN

Confidence intervals consist of a sample mean ± the standard error of the mean (SEM) multiplied by a certain factor. Consider the example of adult height. Imagine selecting a sample of 100 adult males and measuring their heights. On the basis of these 100 measurements, the sample mean and the sample SD can be calculated. Then, on the basis of the SD and the size of the sample (N), the SEM can be calculated as shown in Equation 8.1. Imagine the following hypothetical data:

- $N = 100$
- Mean = 70 inches
- SD = 3.5 inches

The SEM is calculated as:

Equation 8.1:

$$\text{SEM} = \frac{\text{SD}}{\sqrt{N}}$$

$$\text{That is: } \frac{3.5}{10} = 0.35 \text{ inches}$$

As noted at the beginning of this section, CIs are calculated as the mean plus or minus the SEM multiplied by a certain factor. In the case of the commonly employed 95% CI, that factor is 2.0. This value of 2.0 derives from the statement in Section 6.8.1 that 95% of the data points in a Normal distribution fall within ±2 SDs of the mean. (Note that while the multiplicative factor of 2 in the case of the 95% CI is directly related to the statement that 95% of the data points in a Normal distribution fall within ± 2 SDs of the mean, the SEM, and not the SD, is used for purposes of calculating CIs.) Hence

$$95\% \text{ CI} = 70 \pm 2 \text{ SEM} = 70 \pm 0.7 = 69.3\text{–}70.7 \text{ inches.}$$

This range is often written in the form (69.3, 70.7).

8.3.1 A More Precise Definition of a Confidence Interval

The 95% CI is often incorrectly conceptualized as stating that the "real" population mean has a 95% chance of being in the range represented by the lower and upper limits of the CI. In the example used in the previous paragraph, this equates to a statement that the population mean has a 95% chance of lying in the range of

69.3–70.7 inches. Strictly, this is not a meaningful statement: Even though we do not know what it is, the population mean does exist as a precise value, and precise values cannot meaningfully be associated with a probability. In strict terms, the CI is a range of values that is likely to cover the true but unknown population mean (Campbell and Machin, 1999).

8.4 CONFIDENCE INTERVALS FOR THE DIFFERENCE BETWEEN TREATMENT GROUP MEANS

Throughout this book, the usual example employed is a parallel group, randomized clinical trial in which a drug is compared to a placebo. To examine the effects of the treatments over time, a baseline measurement is taken, followed by a measurement at some specified time later. A change score is then calculated for each subject. The fundamental analysis that addresses the drug's efficacy is one in which the mean change in the drug treatment group is compared with the mean change in the placebo treatment group. That is, we are interested in the difference between the means of two treatment groups.

Based on a single study, a 95% CI can be calculated for the difference between the means of two treatment groups, just as it can for the mean of a single parameter such as height (the computation is more complex, but the principle is the same). The difference between the treatment group means is a single value, just like the single value that represents the sample mean height in the example in Section 8.3. The interpretation of CIs for the difference between treatment group means is, in essence, the same as the interpretation of the CI for a single mean. Consider a randomized clinical trial evaluating a new antihypertensive drug. Imagine that the difference between the drug treatment group mean changes (the effect size) was 10 mmHg, and the SEM was 1 mmHg. The 95% CI would then be 10 ± 2SE, or 8–12, typically written as (8, 12). In this case, this CI is a range of values that is likely to cover the true but unknown population effect size.

While the 95% CI is commonly employed in this context, it is also possible to calculate other CIs. For example, another CI of interest is the 99% CI. Recall that CIs are calculated as the mean plus or minus the SEM multiplied by a certain factor. In this case, that factor is 2.576. This value derives from the statement in Section 6.8.1 that 99% of the data points in a Normal distribution fall within ±2.576 SDs of the mean. Note that this value is larger than the multiplication factor for the 95% CI, i.e., 1.960 (often rounded, as noted, to 2.0). Therefore, for any given set of data, the value that is added to and subtracted from the group difference to yield the lower and upper limits of the CI will be greater in the case of the 99% CI than it will be in the case of the 95% CI. This in turn means that the 99% CI will have a larger range than the 95% CI. It is not surprising that, in order to be 99% confident that a range will cover the true but unknown population effect size, this range needs to be larger than a range that you can be 95% confident will cover the true but unknown population effect size.

8.5 Relationship of the 95% CI and 99% CI to the 0.05 and 0.01 p-Values

It has been shown that the $p<0.05$ and the $p<0.01$ significance levels represent two degrees of compelling evidence that a given result did not occur by chance alone. These widely accepted significance levels represent particular degrees of certainty that the treatment groups differ from each other. There are two aspects to the relationship between p-values and CIs. First, it is reasonable to think that the $p<0.05$ significance level and the 95% CI may be related in that the $p<0.05$ level is also called the "5% significance level" and that 5% plus 95% equals 100%. Similarly, it is reasonable to think that the $p<0.01$ significance level and the 99% CI may be related in that the $p<0.01$ level is also called the "1% significance level" and that 1% plus 99% equals 100%.

More importantly, CIs are intimately related to probability levels in that levels of statistical significance can be deduced from the values of the CI limits. For the type of hypothesis testing that we have focused on so far, i.e., examining the difference between the treatment group mean change scores, if the 95% CI excludes zero, the difference will attain significance at the $p<0.05$ level. Similarly, in the case of 99% CIs, if a 99% CI does not contain zero, the difference will attain significance at the $p<0.01$ level. This relationship between CIs and probability levels arises from the fact that, in the scenario of interest here—the possible difference in response for two treatment groups—the "null value" is zero. That is, the effect size that would result if the two group means were identical is zero. Thus, if the 95% CI excludes zero, there is compelling evidence at the 5% level that the effect size is not zero, which means that there is compelling evidence that the treatment group means differ. If the 99% CI excludes zero, there is compelling evidence at the 1% level that the effect size is not zero, which means that there is even stronger evidence that the treatment group means differ.

8.6 The Additional Benefit of Using Confidence Intervals

As just seen, CIs can be used to deduce levels of statistical significance: They do not yield precise p-values, but they can show whether or not a given level of statistical significance is attained. They can therefore be informative in determining whether or not statistical significance is attained. However, they are also uniquely informative in assessing clinical importance: As was noted in Section 8.1, p-values alone cannot do this. Therefore, CIs offer a tremendous advantage over p-values in the clinical context, and they are therefore extremely important in new drug development.

8.6.1 Clinical Relevance and Clinically Relevant Differences

The process of determining clinical relevance is not as straight-forward as determining statistical significance. For any set of data, statistical significance can be evaluated by following the procedural rules of hypothesis testing. However, in clinical research the assessment of clinical relevance is more informative than assessment of statistical significance alone. Consider the example of blood pressure. In practice, antihypertensive therapy is largely, and successfully, based around certain "milestones" that represent delineation between normal blood pressure and elevated blood pressure. While such guidelines are an essential pragmatic component of therapy decisions, there is an added degree of complexity in this case. Based on actuarial data, the relationship between blood pressure and life expectancy is reasonably linear and incremental, in that any increase in blood pressure is associated with a decrease in life expectancy. Therefore, any decrease, no matter how small, is ideologically desirable. However, the practicalities of large- scale pharmacotherapy are greatly assisted by the development of drugs that have "worthwhile" efficacy, since all drugs have side effects too.

Therefore, in terms of the development of a new antihypertensive drug, a question that arises is: What is the minimum mean decrease in SBP in early clinical trials that makes continued development of this drug worthwhile? If such a trial shows that the difference between the drug treatment group mean and the placebo treatment group mean is 3 mmHg, is continued development desirable? In the real world, there are both clinical and commercial considerations that contribute to the answer to the last question. The drug may reliably lower SBP by 3 mmHg, but does this benefit outweigh any potential side effects? Also, if there are other antihypertensive drugs already on the market that safely lower SBP by 3 mmHg or more, would this drug have any chance of being successful in the market even if it were to be approved by the regulatory agency?

In this example of a group difference of 3 mmHg, development would probably not continue. However, at what point would a decision to continue likely be made? This leads to another question: What is the smallest effect size that is clinically meaningful, or clinically relevant? This effect size can be called the clinically relevant difference (CRD). Its determination is a clinical one, not a statistical one. This determination may well be strongly influenced by existing empirical evidence (for example, actuarial statistics), but, unlike statistical significance, its determination is not simply formulaic.

For illustrative purposes here, assume that the CRD is 6 mmHg. That is, if the mean SBP change in the drug treatment group is 6 mmHg or more greater than the mean change in the placebo treatment group, i.e., the effect size is 6 mmHg or greater, the effect size is considered clinically relevant. Clinical relevance is meaningfully evaluated by CIs. Imagine a randomized clinical trial in which the effect size was 10 mmHg and the 95% CI was (8, 12). First, consider the statistical significance of this result. Since the lower and upper limits of the CI exclude zero, the difference between the treatment groups is significant at the $p<0.05$ level. Second, consider the clinical significance of this result. A 95% CI of (8, 12) is a range of values that is likely to cover the true but unknown population effect size. We therefore have compelling evidence from our single trial that the drug would lower SBP between 8 mmHg and 12 mmHg in the general population. Since both of these values are greater than our CRD of 6 mmHg, there is compelling evidence that the drug would be useful in the general population of hypertensives.

In contrast, imagine a randomized clinical trial in which the effect size was 10 mmHg, the same size as in the previous example, and the 95% CI was (5, 15). Since the lower and upper limits of the CI exclude zero, this result is also significant at the $p<0.05$ level. However, the implications for clinical significance are quite different. A 95% CI of (5, 15) is a range of values that is likely to cover the true but unknown population effect size. We therefore have compelling evidence from our single trial that the drug would lower SBP between 5 mmHg and 15 mmHg in the general population. The upper limit of the CI (15 mmHg) is higher than in the previous example, meaning that, based on the results from this single trial, it is possible that the drug could have greater efficacy. However, the more pertinent fact is that the lower limit of 5 mmHg is not only lower than in the previous example, meaning that the drug could have less efficacy, but it is also lower than the CRD value of 6 mmHg. Therefore, based on the results from this single trial, it is possible that this drug would not be clinically useful in hypertensives in general.

As a final example here, consider the implications of the results from a randomized clinical trial in which the effect size was 3 mmHg and the 95% CI was (2, 4). Again, these CI values confirm that the treatment group mean and the placebo group mean change differed statistically significantly from each other, since the lower and upper limits of the CI exclude zero. However, since neither the lower nor the upper limit of the CI is greater than 6 mmHg, there is no evidence to suggest that the drug would be clinically useful in the general population. Statistical significance, therefore, is not in itself a reliable indicator of clinical significance. In these three examples, the effect size attained statistical significance at the 5% level on all three occasions, but the clinical significance of the results in the examples were all different. For this reason it has become highly advisable to report CIs in addition to reporting the results of hypothesis testing in regulatory documentation and clinical publications.

9

SAMPLE-SIZE ESTIMATION

9.1 INTRODUCTION

Sample-size estimation is the process by which a researcher decides how many subjects to include in a given clinical trial. It was noted in Chapter 5 that sample-size estimation is a critical part of the design of clinical trials, and, like all design issues, this must be addressed in the study protocol before the trial commences. However, discussion of this topic was intentionally delayed until this point in the book so that you could read the intervening chapters and acquire an understanding of important concepts, including statistical significance and clinical significance, before reading about sample-size estimation. Addressing sample-size estimation at this point also allows a whole (if short) chapter to be dedicated to this topic, thereby acknowledging its importance in clinical research.

Many sources use the terms "sample-size determination" or "sample-size calculation" when discussing this issue. This book uses the term sample-size estimation to emphasize that deciding on the sample size that will be employed in a clinical trial is a process of estimation that involves both statistical and clinical informed judgment and not a process of simply calculating the "right" answer. It is true that mathematical calculations are made in this process, and, for a given set of values that are placed into the appropriate formula in any given circumstance, a precise answer will be given. However, the values that are placed into the formula are chosen by the sponsor.

Some of the values that need to be entered into the formula are typically chosen from a standard set of possibilities, with the researcher deciding which of several generally acceptable values is best suited for the intentions of a given trial. Other values are estimates based on data that may be available in existing literature or may have been collected in an earlier trial in the clinical development program. These include the estimated treatment effect and the variability associated with the estimated treatment effect. Deciding upon the sample size for a given clinical trial is a balancing act in which several factors need to be considered to achieve the balance desired by the sponsor.

The likelihood of a successful outcome (at least from the point of view that "success" means obtaining a statistically significant result) can be increased by increasing the sample size. When designing a study, the researcher wants to ensure that a large enough sample size is chosen to be able to detect an important difference that does in fact exist. It is certainly possible that a trial can fail to demonstrate such a difference simply because the sample size chosen was too small. Therefore, it might appear reasonable to think that a very big sample size is a good idea. However, there are ethical issues that must be considered when choosing the sample size (see the following section). Additionally, increasing the sample size increases the expenses, difficulties, and overall length of a trial. Somewhere, for each sponsor and each study, an acceptable sample size needs to be chosen that balances the likelihood of a statistically significant result with the cost and time involved in conducting the clinical trial. Indeed, some sponsors have proposed decision-making models to estimate the ideal sample size incorporating various factors such as the length of the study, the financial costs, and usual statistical considerations (see Pallay, 2000).

9.2 ETHICAL ISSUES IN SAMPLE-SIZE ESTIMATION

As discussed in Section 1.8.1, one of the key elements in conducting an ethical clinical trial is the principle of beneficence. This principle requires that the study design is scientifically sound and that any risks of the research are acceptable in relation to the likely benefits from the study. In the context of our present discussions, the phrase "requires that the study design is scientifically sound" is particularly pertinent. As noted in the Foreword to this book, research subjects voluntarily take part in clinical trials not for their personal gain but for the greater good. They are told that that their participation will provide information that is useful and generalizable to a much larger group of people. This is one of the benefits that are weighed against the risks of being exposed to a drug under development. If the design of the trial is such that the data collected do not permit the best possible information to be obtained, the subjects' expectations have been violated.

Sample-size estimation therefore has an important ethical component. There are ethical issues involved in recruiting both too few and too many subjects (Matthews, 2006). Recruiting too few subjects means that the study may be underpowered and unable to detect a treatment effect of interest that actually exists. Such a design is scientifically inadequate to answer the research question of interest (i.e., to address the primary objective of the trial). It is also unethical. Subjects may have taken part in a study that did not have a chance of detecting a treatment effect that may have existed, and thus their expectation that participation may add to the knowledge base about the investigational drug was violated.

It is also unethical to recruit many more subjects than were actually necessary to provide an answer to the research question. Imagine a trial testing a new drug against a placebo in which an answer to the research question could have been obtained with 1,000 subjects (500 in each treatment group). That is, after 1,000 subjects had participated, there could have been compelling evidence that the new drug was safe and more effective than the placebo. If 2,000 subjects actually took part in the trial, one-half of the second thousand subjects would have received the placebo. That is, 500 subjects would have been given a treatment that was inferior. Asking subjects to participate in clinical trials in which a new drug is evaluated against a control drug is only ethical if there is no existing evidence at that time that the new drug is more effective (recall the discussion of clinical equipoise in Section 1.8.1).

Sample-size estimation therefore takes on a special significance in clinical trials. As noted in Section 9.1, this process of estimation does not produce the "right" answer, so it is not possible to specify precisely what constitutes "too few" or "too many" subjects. However, it is imperative to estimate a reasonable sample size based on the best evidence that is available at the time and with full knowledge of the implications of this estimate.

9.3 VARIABLES INVOLVED IN SAMPLE-SIZE ESTIMATION

Several variables need to be considered in the process of sample-size estimation. The values of these variables in any given case can be chosen by the sponsor based on several considerations. Some terms that will be useful for present discussions are:

- Type I errors and Type II errors. As noted in Section 7.10.1, a Type I error occurs when a significant result is "found" when it does not really exist, and a Type II error occurs when one fails to find a significant difference that actually exists.
- The probability of making a Type I error, α. This is also the level of statistical significance chosen, typically 0.05, but it is possible to choose 0.01 or even more conservative values.
- The probability of making a Type II error, β. As discussed in Section 6.5, a probability value must be between 0 and 1: therefore, β will be between 0 and 1.
- Power, calculated as 1 minus β. Since the probability represented by β will be between 0 and 1, power will also be between 0 and 1 since it is defined as 1 minus β. In the context of our ongoing example of developing a new antihypertensive, the power of a trial describes its ability to find a difference between treatment groups when such a difference actually exists. As noted in Section 5.5.3, the power of a statistical test is the probability that the null hypothesis is rejected when it is indeed false. Since rejecting the null hypothesis when it is false is extremely desirable, it is generally regarded that the power of a study should be as great as practically feasible.
- An estimation of the treatment effect. This is usually the difference between means or proportions. In this book's ongoing example involving a new investigative antihypertensive drug, the treatment effect is the difference between the mean drug treatment group SBP response and the mean placebo treatment group SBP response.
- An estimation of the variance in the treatment effect (the standard deviation is typically used here).
- The standardized treatment effect, calculated by dividing the estimated treatment effect by its estimated standard deviation.
- The sample size, *N*, that is provided by the calculation performed using the values chosen by the researcher.

9.4 TYPE I AND TYPE II ERRORS

Type I and Type II errors were introduced in Section 7.10.1. In the context of this book's ongoing example involving a new investigative antihypertensive drug, a Type I error occurs when a significant difference between treatment groups is found when it does not really exist. This occurrence is also known as a false-positive finding. A Type II error occurs when the sponsor fails to find a significant difference that does actually exist, an occurrence also known as a false negative. (It should be noted here that different types of study designs, such as the equivalence and noninferiority designs discussed in Chapter 11, require different types of null hypotheses and different expressions of Type I and Type II errors. They also require different formulas for sample-size estimation. This chapter's discussions address the book's ongoing example involving the development of a new antihypertensive drug.)

Setting β at 0.10 means that the sponsor is willing to accept a 10% chance of missing an association of a given treatment effect size (the treatment effect size chosen by the sponsor). That is, the sponsor is willing to accept a 10% chance of a Type II error occurring. Put the other way, this means that there is a 90% chance of finding a treatment effect of the magnitude chosen (or greater) for the sample-size estimation. Thus, in 9 out of 10 studies (90%), the investigator would likely be able to correctly reject the null hypothesis (given that the assumed standard deviation is correct).

Table 9.1 provides a concise picture of the implications of false-positive findings and false-negative findings. One of two actions—rejecting the null hypothesis or failing to reject the null hypothesis—must occur at the end of all hypothesis testing, and the action taken is determined by the significance of the test statistic obtained in the statistical analysis conducted. If the test statistic attains statistical significance, the sponsor rejects the null hypothesis; if the test statistic does not attain statistical significance, the sponsor fails to reject the null hypothesis.

Table 9.1. Type I Errors and Type II Errors

	Reality	
Action Based on Study Results	Research Hypothesis Is True	Null Hypothesis Is True
Reject null hypothesis	Correct action	Type I error (false positive)
Fail to reject null hypothesis	Type II error (false negative)	Correct action

9.4.1 The Implications of Type I and Type II Errors

Table 9.1 shows that the results from a clinical trial can lead the sponsor to an inappropriate conclusion in some cases. In these cases, one of two types of error occurs:

- Type I error (false-positive): In this scenario, the sponsor rejects the null hypothesis, e.g., "finds" a statistically significant difference between the drug treatment group mean response and the placebo treatment group mean response in the type of study used in our ongoing example of an antihypertensive drug. The inference from this finding, based on the sample of subjects employed in this trial, is that the drug would be effective in the population from which the sample was chosen.
- Type II error (false-negative): In this case, the sponsor fails to reject the null hypothesis, i.e., fails to find a statistically significant difference between the drug treatment group mean response and the placebo treatment group mean response. The inference from this finding, based on the sample of subjects employed in this trial, is that the drug would not be effective in the population from which the sample was chosen.

Ideally, the likelihood of either type of error would be zero, or at least as low as possible. In reality, the possibility of making these errors cannot totally be eliminated, but their likely occurrence can be balanced one against the other. This is done by choosing various combinations of α and β, and therefore various combinations of α and power, since power is defined as 1 minus β.

9.5 CHOOSING THE VARIABLES NEEDED FOR SAMPLE-SIZE ESTIMATION

As noted in Section 9.1, several variables are needed for sample-size estimation, and the researcher can choose the values to be used in the formula that will yield the sample size, *N*. These are α, β, the estimated treatment effect, and its variance.

9.5.1 Alpha and Beta

The estimation of a sample size requires several variables to be chosen. In each case, the following need to be selected:

- The significance level (α), usually 0.05. Choosing $\alpha = 0.05$ means that on 95% of occasions the null hypothesis will be rejected correctly. That is, the researcher is willing to accept a 5% chance that a positive finding will result by chance alone. Generally, regulatory agencies are concerned about Type I (false-positive) errors: They do not want to grant marketing approval on the basis of erroneously favorable data. This occurrence is made acceptably low by typically choosing $\alpha = 0.05$ and sometimes choosing $\alpha = 0.01$ to be really conservative.

- Adequate power. In the context of our ongoing example, power is the ability of a study to find a difference between treatment groups when such a difference actually exists. Power is calculated as 1 minus β. In most clinical trials, adequate power is regarded as at least 80%, and it is typically 90%. In contrast to regulatory agencies' concern with Type I errors, sponsors are generally concerned about Type II (false-negative) errors: They do not want to erroneously conclude that their drug does not work by obtaining a nonsignificant result when the drug does actually work. Doing this will likely result in the drug not being brought to market when it might have been. So, sponsors want enough power to detect a real difference when it exists, i.e., to reject the null hypothesis when it should be rejected. So, ideally, they probably want (at least) 90% power. Selecting 90% power sets β at 0.10, since power equals 1 minus β.

9.5.2 The Treatment Effect, Its Variance, and the Standardized Treatment Effect

For the ongoing example in this book, i.e., testing a new antihypertensive drug against a placebo control, the following values must also be chosen:

- The clinically relevant difference (CRD) that the test is required to detect. This is the treatment effect size, i.e., the difference between the mean drug treatment group response and the mean placebo treatment group response, that the sponsor deems clinically relevant.
- The standard deviation (SD) of the treatment effect.
- The standardized effect size, calculated as the ratio CRD/SD.

Determining the clinically relevant difference to look for in the study is relatively straightforward. Another way to conceptualize the clinically relevant difference is as the smallest effect size that is clinically meaningful. This can be based on clinical input. For example, a decrease in SBP of 10 mmHg may be thought by the sponsor to be clinically relevant in this context.

The standard deviation for change in SBP can be harder to determine. One way is to examine previously published data on similar outcomes (maybe other drugs in the same class). If few data are available from this source, consulting with experts in this research domain may be helpful. Another possibility is to conduct a small pilot study. In the later phases of a clinical development program, data from earlier studies may be informative. This often means that for confirmatory clinical drug trials there will be results from earlier trials, so information is readily available. From these two items, the standardized effect size can be calculated as the ratio CRD/SD.

9.6 USING THE APPROPRIATE FORMULA TO YIELD THE SAMPLE SIZE

Sample-size estimation can be performed for any study design. In each case, the respective formula will be used to estimate the sample size required (see Chow et al., 2003). For the formula used in the type of study design that we are using as our ongoing example, each of the variables we have discussed will have certain influences on the sample size, *N*, that will be given by the formula. These influences, i.e., their relationships with *N* given that all of the others remain the same, can be summarized as follows:

- The smaller the chosen value of α, the larger the value of *N* that will be given.
- The smaller the chosen value of β, the larger the value of *N* that will be given. This is because power is defined as 1 minus β. As β decreases, power increases; as power increases, the larger the value of *N* that will be given.
- The larger the standardized effect size, the smaller the value of *N* that will be given.

The third of these relationships, the relationship between standardized effect size and *N*, is actually influenced by the two separate factors that determine the standardized effect size once each of these factors has been chosen. As noted in Section 9.5.2, the standardized effect size is calculated as the ratio CRD/SD. Since the CRD is the numerator in this ratio, the larger the CRD, the larger the standardized effect size will be for a given SD. And, conversely, since SD is the denominator in the ratio, the larger the SD, the smaller the standardized effect size will be for a given CRD. Therefore, the larger the SD, the larger the *N* that will be given by the sample-size estimation.

9.7 INFLUENCES ON THE SPONSOR'S CHOICE OF THESE VALUES

As we have discussed, when conducting a sample-size estimation, the researcher has to choose values for α and β and has to come up with a standardized treatment effect, which is in turn the result of finding the best possible estimates of a clinically significant difference and its variation. What are the influences that lead the sponsor to choose certain values for α, β, and the standardized treatment effect?

For financial, time demand, and logistical reasons, a smaller sample size is preferable to a sponsor than a larger one. There are also ethical factors that need to be borne in mind. It is unethical to choose a sample that can reasonably be considered either too small or too large (see Section 9.2). The optimum sample size can be considered to be the smallest sample size that can reasonably be expected to answer the primary research question, i.e., evaluating the primary objective as stated in the study protocol.

What might influence the sponsor's choice of α and β? It was noted in Section 9.5.1 that a typical value for α is 0.05 and a typical value for β is 0.10 (i.e., a typical power is 90%). Circumstances in which it may make sense to choose different values include the following:

- For a drug with nasty side effects, it will be necessary to have particularly compelling evidence that it is effective. That is, it will be necessary to demonstrate highly statistically significant efficacy, and there is a strong need to avoid false-positive results, i.e., to avoid a Type I error. Therefore, the sponsor will likely set α lower than usual, perhaps at 0.01 or even 0.001. This choice of α being set at lower than the typical 0.05 will result in a greater N being given by the sample-size estimation.
- If a study is particularly difficult to repeat, and therefore the trial being planned is the sponsor's "one shot" at getting relevant data, it is a good idea to give the study as much power as is practically possible. So, the sponsor may increase the study's power to a higher value than usual. Since power is calculated as 1 minus β, the sponsor needs to reduce β in order to increase the study's power, which means that the chance of a Type II error, i.e., not finding a treatment effect that actually exists, is reduced. This choice of β as lower than the typical 0.10 will result in a greater N being given by the sample-size estimation.
- If the sponsor is conducting a study early in product development and wishes to optimize power on that occasion while "compromising" α, β might be chosen as 0.10 and α as 0.10 or even 0.15 or 0.20 (Donahue and Ruberg, 1997).

While either action, i.e., reducing α or β, will increase the value of N given by the sample-size estimation and therefore result in additional cost to the sponsor, the sponsor may well decide that, in the overall balancing act of estimating sample size, there are good reasons to do this in cases such as these examples.

At each stage of the drug development program and for each trial within that stage, sponsors need to be aware of the implications of their choice of α and their choice of β and the acceptability of these implications. The implications of each choice and the acceptability of these implications may change throughout the course of a clinical development program.

9.8 CHOOSING THE OBJECTIVE(S) ON WHICH TO BASE THE SAMPLE-SIZE ESTIMATION

A sample-size estimation must be based on a specific objective in a clinical trial's study protocol. By the time sample-size estimation becomes particularly meaningful, i.e., in later-stage clinical trials designed to demonstrate efficacy, it is a very good idea to have a single objective (the primary objective) and a single identifiable endpoint or outcome of interest. In this case, the sample-size estimation is based on this objective. However, this situation is not always the case, and more than one outcome measure is regarded as equally important by the researcher. In these situations, a common approach is to conduct the sample-size estimates for each outcome measure and then select the largest of these as the sample size required to answer all the questions of interest (Machin and Campbell, 2005).

This approach, however, raises issues of multiplicity (see Section 7.10). Accordingly, lower p-values may be required to be able to declare a result as statistically significant. This means that an adjustment to the sample-size estimation formula is appropriate, with the precise nature of the adjustment being related to the number of outcomes to be tested. This adjustment raises the magnitude of the estimated sample size (Machin and Campbell, 2005).

9.9 Other Issues to Keep in Mind

It is useful to keep several other issues in mind when conducting sample-size estimations, including the following:

- Possible attrition. It is likely that all of the subjects that start a clinical trial will not complete it. This attrition may increase with the demands of a trial (e.g., number of clinic visits required, degree of discomfort caused by any procedures or measurements). It is important to consider the possible (likely) attrition rate when estimating the number of subjects needed for the "successful" analysis of the data, and to increase the number chosen appropriately.
- Overly optimistic choice of treatment effect. As Machin and Campbell (2005) noted in the context of comparative clinical trials, researchers "are often optimistic about the magnitude of the improvement of the new treatments over the standard." Since a larger estimated treatment effect leads to a smaller sample size being chosen, overestimating the estimated treatment effect may lead to a smaller but still clinically important effect not being detected, since the sample size adopted was too small to detect it.
- In some instances (e.g., late-stage development) the sample size required is driven not by statistical considerations for demonstrating effect but by minimal exposure requirements for safety considerations (see ICH Guideline E1).

Part IV

Lifecycle Clinical Development

10

Safety Assessment in Clinical Trials

10.1 Introduction

The safety of a drug is addressed at all stages in its life history: discovery and design, nonclinical research, clinical development, and postmarketing surveillance. As noted in Chapter 3, *in silico* modeling in the discovery phase of synthetic drugs can examine the potential interactions of centers of reactivity in a drug with non-target receptors, interactions that can lead to undesirable effects. Such studies are intended to modify the eventual drug molecule in a beneficial manner, thereby enhancing its safety profile. Safety evaluation in nonclinical research was discussed in Chapter 4. Discussions of safety in this part of the book, Lifecycle Clinical Development, focus on the involvement of human subjects in (experimental) clinical trials (this chapter) and then on nonexperimental large-scale evaluations of an approved drug in general use (Chapter 13).

Before discussing safety assessment in clinical trials, an overview of clinical trials is presented. This is pertinent to the discussion of safety data in this chapter and also to the discussion of efficacy data collected in clinical trials that follows in Chapter 11.

10.2 Classification of Clinical Trials

Pharmaceutical clinical trials are often categorized into various phases, with any given trial being identified as belonging to one of them. These categories include Phase I, Phase II, and Phase III, and this common nomenclature was employed in Chapter 1 since it is likely that you were already familiar with it. However, there are alternate systems of categorization that are arguably more informative. A "traditional" description of phases is as follows:

- Phase I trials. Pharmacologically oriented studies that typically look for the best dose to employ. Comparison to other treatments is not typically built into the study design.
- Phase II trials. Trials that look for evidence of activity, efficacy, and safety at a fixed dose. Comparison to other treatments is not typically built into the study design.
- Phase III trials. Trials in which comparison with another treatment (e.g., placebo, an active control) is a fundamental component of the design. These trials are undertaken if Phase I and Phase II studies have provided preliminary evidence that the new treatment is safe and effective.

New Drug Development: Design, Methodology, and Analysis. By J. Rick Turner

Other phase designations have also become employed in various areas, including Phase IIa, Phase IIb, and Phase IIIb (see Buncher and Tsay, 2006a). However, these designations are not used consistently. Therefore, two studies with the same aims may be classified into different phases, and two studies classified into the same phase may have different aims. This nomenclature, therefore, can be confusing. An alternative system has been suggested by the ICH.

10.2.1. Descriptive Terminology as Suggested by ICH

As shown in Table 10.1, ICH Guideline E8 provides an approach to classifying clinical studies according to their objective. This book therefore presents subsequent discussions of clinical trials using the descriptive terminology suggested by the ICH.

10.3 THE WIDE VARIETY OF CLINICAL ASSESSMENTS CONDUCTED

A multitude of studies are conducted to examine the safety and efficacy of a new investigational drug in humans. Among the goals of clinical development are the following:

- Estimation of the investigational drug's safety and tolerance in healthy adults.
- Determination of a safe and effective dose range, safe dosing levels, and the preferred route of administration.
- Investigation of pharmacokinetics and pharmacodynamics following a single-dose and a multiple-dose schedule.
- Establishment and validation of biochemical markers in accessible body fluids that may permit the assessment of the desired pharmacological activity.
- Identification of metabolic pathways.
- Evaluation of the drug's safety and efficacy in a relatively small group of subjects with the disease or condition of interest (the targeted therapeutic indication).
- Optimization and then selection of final formulations, doses, regimens, and efficacy endpoints for larger scale, multicenter studies. Efficacy endpoints should be able to be measured reliably and should quantitatively reflect clinically relevant changes in the disease or condition of interest.
- Evaluation of the drug's comparative efficacy (with placebo or an active comparator) in larger scale, multicenter studies and collection of additional safety data.

Additional safety data and effectiveness data (see Chapter 13) are collected in therapeutic use studies. The following statement by Piantadosi (2005) is particularly salient here:

Table 10.1. Classifying Clinical Studies According to Their Objectives

Objective of Study	Study Examples
Human Pharmacology •Assess tolerance. •Describe or define pharmacokinetics (PK) and pharmacodynamics (PD). •Explore drug metabolism and drug interactions. •Estimate (biological) activity.	•Dose-tolerance studies. •Single- and multiple-dose PK and/or PD studies. •Drug interaction studies.
Therapeutic Exploratory •Explore use for the targeted indication. •Estimate dosage for subsequent studies. •Provide basis for confirmatory study design, endpoints, methodologies.	•Earliest trials of relatively short duration in well-defined narrow patient populations, using surrogate of pharmacological endpoints or clinical measures. •Dose-response exploration studies.
Therapeutic Confirmatory •Demonstrate/confirm efficacy. •Establish safety profile. •Provide an adequate basis for assessing benefit/risk relationship to support licensing. •Establish dose-response relationship.	•Adequate and well-ontrolled studies to establish efficacy. •Randomized parallel dose-response studies. •Clinical safety studies. •Studies of mortality/morbidity outcomes. •Large simple trials. •Comparative studies.
Therapeutic Use •Refine understanding of benefit/risk relationship in general or special populations and/or environments. •Identify less common adverse reactions. •Refine dosing recommendation.	•Comparative effectiveness studies. •Studies of mortality/morbidity outcomes. •Studies of additional endpoints. •Large simple trials. •Pharmacoeconomic studies.

From ICH E8: General Considerations for Clinical Trials.

> A trialist must understand two different modes of thinking that support the science—clinical and statistical. They both underlie the re-emergence of therapeutics as a modern science. Each method of reasoning arose independently and must be combined skillfully if they are to serve therapeutic questions effectively (p.10).

The chapters in this part of the book discuss both clinical and statistical issues and illustrate how they are combined together for the ultimate benefit of patients.

10.4 HUMAN PHARMACOLOGY TRIALS

The commencement of human pharmacology clinical trials (FTIH trials) can lead to a range of emotions for clinical researchers. It is a time of excitement (and quite possibly relief) that the drug has reached this milestone and a time of anticipation and hopeful expectation. Additionally, and possibly more so, it is a time of trepidation and anxiousness. As noted in Section 4.5, no animal model is a perfect predictor of the precise effects of the drug in humans, and there is the ever present possibility that serious safety issues may arise. On relatively rare occasions, life-threatening, drug-induced conditions have occurred in subjects in human pharmacology clinical trials.

The main objectives in human pharmacology studies are to assess the safety of the drug, to obtain a thorough knowledge and understanding of the drug's pharmacokinetic profile and potential interactions with other drugs, and to estimate pharmacodynamic activity. A range of doses and/or dosing intervals is investigated in a sequential manner. Characterization of the drug's safety profile may include investigation of pharmacokinetics, structure-activity relationships, mechanisms of action, and identifying preferred routes of administration and interactions with other medications. A well-conducted human pharmacology study can reduce the possibility of later failed trials.

Typically, between 20 and 80 healthy adults (this number can certainly be lower) participate in these relatively short studies, and subjects are often recruited from university medical school settings where trials are being conducted. Subjects are typically paid for their participation. (This payment may be one reason why the term "volunteers" originated to describe these subjects—see the discussion in Section 1.8.2. However, there are financial benefits to many clinical trial participants in later clinical trials too, in that medical procedures involved in trials are conducted at no cost to the subjects.)

During human pharmacology studies, subjects are given extensive physical examinations before the administration of the drug, after its administration, and, in the case of longer term studies, at various intervals throughout the treatment. An extensive battery of typical tests includes:

- Liver function.
- Kidney function.
- Blood chemistry.
- Urine chemistry.
- Eye testing.
- Others specific to target organ systems.

Human pharmacology studies are designed to collect data that can be compared with similar types of data collected in nonclinical studies. Acute single-dose studies are conducted first, with the dose used based on extrapolation from nonclinical work. Short-term studies of various doses follow, and then longer-term studies of various doses are conducted. Eventually, dose-finding studies are conducted to determine the maximum tolerated dose (MTD) of the drug. These studies facilitate the examination of pharmacokinetic parameters and toxicity. They are designed to answer questions concerning the side effects that are seen, their characteristics, and whether they are consistent to any notable degree across subjects (see Chevret, 2006, for more details).

From a statistical viewpoint, the design of these studies has certain implications. They include a relatively small number of subjects, but a lot of measurements are collected for each subject. This strategy has both advantages and limitations. The extensive array of measurements made allows the drug's effects to be characterized reasonably thoroughly. However, because so few subjects participate in these studies, generalizations to the general subject population are relatively harder than for studies with larger sample sizes. This observation may be particularly pertinent in the case of dose-finding MTD studies.

10.5 THERAPEUTIC EXPLORATORY STUDIES

Trials focusing on comprehensive assessment of an investigational drug's safety in a relatively small group of subjects with the disease or condition of interest are typically conducted by clinical pharmacologists. These trials often involve hospitalized subjects who can be closely monitored. These trials include both subjective self-report assessments by the subjects and (more) objective biochemical assessments, e.g., change in liver enzymes. Trials that examine efficacy in similar groups of subjects are typically conducted by individuals specifically trained in clinical trial methodology and execution. Some authors have voiced the opinion that these trials provide the most accurate assessment of efficacy, since they are conducted in a very tightly controlled manner.

However, in one of the interesting twists that are involved in the comprehensive assessment of a drug's suitability for use by a large target population, other authors note that, while the very tight experimental methodology that is possible in these studies very likely means that this is true, this environment is not typical of the environments in which the drug will eventually be used if approved. The characteristics of later studies in the clinical development program address this issue. First, therapeutic confirmatory trials are typically multicenter trials that are conducted in an environment that is closer to those in which the drug will eventually be used if approved. Second, large-scale assessments that are conducted once the drug has been approved and is being used by a large number of patients do indeed address the question of "efficacy" in realistic real-world environments. In this context, the term "effectiveness" is typically used. These assessments are discussed in more detail in Chapter 13.

10.6 THERAPEUTIC CONFIRMATORY CLINICAL TRIALS

Human pharmacology and therapeutic exploratory studies define the most likely safe and effective dosage regimens for use in subsequent therapeutic confirmatory studies. These therapeutic confirmatory studies are typically run as double-blind, randomized, concurrently controlled clinical trials.

The technique of randomization was pioneered in the field of agriculture (plants too show considerable individual variation) by Sir Ronald Fisher, a visionary statistician. It is generally acknowledged that the first randomized clinical trial, conducted in the 1940s, was a study evaluating the use of streptomycin in treating tuberculosis conducted by the (British) Medical Research Council Streptomycin in Tuberculosis Trials Committee. The results were published in the *British Medical Journal* in 1948.

Matthews (1999) made the following observation concerning randomized trials:

> Over the last two to three decades randomized concurrently controlled clinical trials have become established as the method which investigators must use to assess new treatments if their claims are to find widespread acceptance. The methodology underpinning these trials is firmly based in statistical theory, and the success of randomized trials perhaps constitutes the greatest achievement of statistics in the second half of the twentieth century (Preface).

The discipline of Statistics is employed in clinical trials to investigate a new drug's safety and efficacy. This investigation may provide compelling evidence that the drug is safe and will induce a biological response that improves patients' well-being.

10.7 THERAPEUTIC USE TRIALS

Therapeutic use investigation of drug safety and efficacy data is discussed in Chapter 13.

10.8 THE TERM "DOSE"

The term dose appears frequently when discussing pharmacological therapy. Although the concept of dose initially appears quite simple, it is not easy to define unequivocally. As Hellman (2006) observed, it can refer to:

- External dose: the amount of drug administered.
- Internal or systemic dose: usually, the concentration in the blood.
- Tissue or organ dose: the amount of the drug actually present at the critical site for a sufficient period of time.

The optimum place to assess the concentration of a drug is in the microenvironment of the target receptor (recall the discussions in Chapter 3). However, given the difficulties involved in measuring concentrations in tissues and organs in human subjects and patients, the systemic dose is used most often since it is the most informative measure that is readily available. Concentrations are usually measured in bodily fluids, including blood, blood plasma, blood serum, saliva, urine, and cerebrospinal fluid, with the assumption that drug concentrations in these fluids are in equilibrium with the drug's concentration at its target receptor (Dhillon and Gill, 2006). A typical form of collecting one of these fluids is from a vein in the nondominant arm. Plasma and serum are both easier to use in this context than blood, which causes interference in many assays, and, additionally, plasma is easier to prepare than serum.

Dosage can be defined as the amount of a drug administered over time, e.g., in repeat dose studies (Hellman, 2006).

10.9 CLINICAL PHARMACOKINETICS AND PHARMACODYNAMICS

Pharmacokinetics can be thought of as the relationship between input and exposure over time, and pharmacodynamics as the relationship between exposure and response over time. Pharmacokinetic/pharmacodynamic modeling combines these relationships into a model that represents a complete picture of the relationship between drug administration and response over time. Discussions in this chapter focus on drugs that are administered orally and act systemically. Drugs act systemically when they are absorbed into the blood and delivered to the site of action by blood circulation. A systemically acting drug is distributed to the various organs of the body by the blood. While not all drugs satisfy both of these criteria, many that do are commonly used in clinical treatment. The following discussions therefore focus on aspects of pharmacokinetics and pharmacodynamics that are pertinent to these drugs. This means that they focus on the pharmacokinetics of orally administered small-molecule drugs: As was noted in Chapter 3, the pharmacokinetics of biopharmaceuticals are different. (See Subrahmanyam and Tonelli, 2005, and Braeckman, 2005, for further discussions of the pharmacokinetics of small molecules and of protein therapeutics, respectively.)

As was noted in Chapter 4, pharmacokinetic and pharmacodynamic effects are studied in nonclinical research. These topics are also of critical importance in clinical investigations. A drug's pharmacokinetics and pharmacodynamics are of considerable interest to clinicians who may prescribe the drug to patients once it is approved. Meaningful decisions about a drug's optimal use can only be made with an understanding of the time course of events that occur after the drug's administration, and both pharmacokinetics and pharmacodynamics are concerned with this time course. By consideration of the pharmacokinetic processes of absorption, distribution, metabolism, and excretion (ADME), the discipline of pharmacokinetics provides a quantitative basis to assess the time course of drugs and drug effects (Dhillon and Gill, 2006).

The disciplines of pharmacokinetics and pharmacodynamics allow the quantification and integration of knowledge concerning a drug's journey through the body (kinetics) and the drug response it gives rise to (dynamics). This integration of information comprises the quantitative basis of drug therapy by addressing questions regarding drug administration, such as how much drug should be given, how often it should be given, and for how long. Quantitative answers to these questions facilitate a rational approach to the establishment, optimization, and individualization of dosage regimens in clinical patients (Tozer and Rowland, 2006).

In both pharmacokinetic and pharmacodynamic considerations, an important emphasis concerns the rate at which events occur and the rate at which circumstances change. The pharmacokinetic phase covers the relationship between drug input and the concentration achieved over time. The pharmacodynamic phase covers the relationship between concentration and the therapeutic effect over time (toxicodynamics is concerned with the relationship between concentration and adverse effects over time).

10.10 PHARMACOKINETIC PARAMETERS

Early clinical studies usually perform pharmacokinetic assessments in fasting subjects, thereby avoiding the possible confounding effects of food. While this methodology has a sound logic in initial studies, some early phase investigation of the effects of food on absorption is also warranted. If knowledge of pharmacokinetics were obtained only from fasting subjects, similar restrictions would be necessary in therapeutic exploratory and therapeutic confirmatory trials.

It was noted in the previous section that both pharmacokinetics and pharmacodynamics are concerned with relationships over time. One illustration of the fundamental importance of the rates of these processes can be seen in the plasma concentration-time profile (also known as the plasma-concentration curve) for an administered drug. This was introduced in Section 4.2.1, along with several quantitative pharmacokinetic terms used to describe and quantify aspects of the plasma concentration-time profile:

- C_{max}: The maximum concentration or maximum systemic exposure.
- T_{max}: The time of maximum concentration or time of maximum exposure.
- $t_{½}$, Half-life: The time required to reduce the plasma concentration to one half of its initial value.
- $AUC_{(0-t)}$, the area under the curve from time zero to time t: A measure of total systemic exposure.

However, while informative, this description is only a starting point. Understanding and prediction are more important than simple description (Rolan and Molnar, 2006). To gain this understanding and predictive ability, additional pharmacokinetic parameters are useful. These include:

- Bioavailability. The proportion of an administered dose that reaches the systemic (whole body) circulation in an unchanged form. This is a different measure from absorption.
- Clearance. The volume of plasma that is cleared of drug per unit time by metabolism and excretion. Clearance is calculated additively: The total clearance is the sum of clearance by the liver, the kidneys, and other routes.
- Elimination. The irreversible loss of drug from the site of measurement. It occurs via two processes, excretion and metabolism. Excretion is the irreversible loss of chemically unchanged drug. Metabolism is the conversion of one drug compound to another.
- Elimination rate constant (k). An elimination rate constant that is used in the calculation of the rate of elimination.
- Disposition. A term that embraces both elimination and distribution.

These parameters all have specific uses in determining important aspects of dosage. Knowledge of bioavailability is useful for determining both loading and maintenance doses for orally administered drugs. Knowledge of clearance (in addition to bioavailability) is useful in determining the maintenance dose necessary to achieve a given plasma concentration of the drug. Knowledge of volume (in addition to bioavailability) is useful in determining the loading dose (Rolan and Molnar, 2006).

10.10.1 Absorption and Bioavailability

The term "absorption" refers to the rate and extent to which an administered dose of a drug is taken into the body. In the case of oral administration, interest lies with the rate and extent of systemic absorption from the gastrointestinal tract following administration. If a drug is taken into the intestinal cells, it is deemed to have been absorbed, regardless of the extent to which it is metabolized. In contrast, the term "bioavailability" refers to the proportion of an administered dose that reaches the systemic circulation unchanged.

Maximum bioavailability results after an intravenous injection. In this case, the bioavailability is by definition 100%. When administered orally, however, a drug experiences first-pass metabolism, also called first-pass loss. The nature of the human body means that orally administered drugs travel via the hepatic portal vein to the liver, the major organ of metabolism, before being circulated systemically. Therefore, before the drug gets a chance to exert any therapeutic activity, it has to withstand this first attack on its integrity. Orally administered agents typically have a bioavailability of less than 100%. The degree of first-pass metabolism for a given drug will be influenced by its chemical and physical properties.

The most rigorous quantitative way to assess the extent of bioavailability for an orally administered drug is to compare the areas under the respective plasma-concentration curves following oral and intravenous administration of the same dose of drug. The AUC is then calculated for both, and a ratio is calculated by dividing the AUC for the oral administration by the AUC for the intravenous administration. If the area ratio for the drug administered orally and intravenously is 0.5 (50%), only 50% of the oral dose was absorbed systemically. The term "relative bioavailability" is used when there are no intravenous AUC data available (for various reasons) for the direct comparison with orally administered AUC data. Relative bioavailability is determined by comparing the fractions of drug absorbed for different dosage forms, routes of administration, and conditions (e.g., with and without food).

While the therapeutic outcomes of low absorption and low availability can be similar (both lead to low concentrations of the drug in the blood), separate investigation and quantification of these factors can be beneficial. For example, a drug that is well absorbed but experiences a very high first-pass metabolism can demonstrate low bioavailability. Low absorption and low bioavailability are likely to be improved in different ways, including chemical modification, reformulation, and changing the route of administration (see Rolan and Molnar, 2006).

10.10.2 Distribution

Most drugs require access to tissues to exert their therapeutic effects. Therefore, when investigating the time course of a drug's action, understanding the rate and extent of transfer from blood plasma to the target tissues is essential. The pharmacokinetic profile can provide quantitative clues indicating that the drug is extensively distributed outside the plasma.

10.10.3 Metabolism

Understanding the metabolism of an investigative drug as early as possible in the clinical development program is important for several reasons, including the following:

- Metabolites that were not seen in nonclinical work may be observed in humans. There will therefore be no toxicology data for these metabolites available from the nonclinical database.
- While nonclinical work can provide clues to potential metabolite activity, data from clinical trials are necessary for quantification of concentrations.
- Prediction of the drug's likely interaction (or lack thereof) with other drugs and drug classes is facilitated by identification of the enzymes that metabolize the drug. If a drug is likely to interact with other drugs, this could be detrimental

to a drug's potential commercial success. If a drug is unlikely to interact with certain other drugs, exclusion criteria in later clinical efficacy trials may not need to specify certain concomitant medications (Rolan and Molnar, 2006).

10.10.4 Elimination and Clearance

Rolan and Molnar (2006) discussed metabolism and excretion together, since both result in the disappearance of the drug from plasma. Studies of clearance can be used to investigate bioavailability, e.g., the influence of food. Knowledge of clearance is very important in establishing a dosing regimen: It is used to predict steady-state concentrations when repeated dosing is employed. Some of the drug development issues that can usefully be addressed by careful consideration of pharmacokinetic data are:

- Is the drug adequately absorbed to elicit a therapeutic effect and is it absorbed at a rate that is consistent with the desired clinical response?
- Does the drug stay in the body long enough to be consistent with the desired duration of action?
- Does a relationship exist between plasma concentrations and a relevant measure of drug effect?
- In terms of ADME profiles, do subsets of the target population behave differently from the general population?
- Having considered these and other issues, what is a suitable dosing regimen for therapeutic exploratory and therapeutic confirmatory trials?

10.11 MECHANISMS OF GENETIC INFLUENCES ON METABOLISM

Metabolism is a complex and fascinating process. It is extremely useful in getting rid of bodily toxicants. Apart from all of the toxicants in the man-made environment around us, even animal and plant food contains many chemicals that have no nutritional value but do have potential toxicity. If these chemicals are sufficiently lipid-soluble, they will reach the blood, and they will not be readily excreted unless they are converted to more water-soluble metabolites. This may be the reason why all animals have a wide variety of xenobiotic-metabolizing enzymes that convert a wide range of chemical structures to water-soluble metabolites that can be excreted in urine (Mulder, 2006).

Humans have a high concentration of xenobiotic-metabolizing enzymes in the gut mucosa and in the liver. This arrangement ensures that systemic exposure to potentially toxic chemicals is limited. A high percentage of these may be caught in first-pass metabolism. However, the normally beneficial first-pass metabolism creates problems in drug therapy, being responsible for the typically less-than-100% bioavailability of most orally administered drugs.

Mulder (2006) noted that drug metabolism can be divided into three phases:

- Phase 1 metabolism. The chemical structure of the compound is modified by oxidation, reduction, or hydrolysis. This process forms an acceptor group.
- Phase 2 metabolism. A chemical group is attached to the acceptor group. This typically generates metabolites that are more water-soluble and are therefore more readily excreted.
- Phase 3 metabolism. Transporters transport the drug or metabolites out of the cell in which Phase 1 and Phase 2 metabolism has occurred.

The focus here is on oxidation in Phase 1 metabolism.

10.11.1 Cytochrome P450 Enzymes

The major oxidative drug-metabolizing pathway is catalyzed by cytochrome P450 enzymes (Mulder, 2006). The abbreviation CYP is typically used in this context. More than 60 CYPs have been identified. These are identified by up to four characters (letters or numbers). For example, in the term CYP2A4*4 the letters and numbers indicate the following:

- CYP: superfamily.
- 2: family.
- A: subfamily.
- 4: isoform.
- *4 (the digit that occurs after the asterisk): A particular mutant form.

Genetic effects between individuals in drug metabolism can be largely explained by genetic influences on drug-metabolizing enzymes. Genetic mutations (point mutations or deletions) occur in enzymes that can result in changes in the enzyme's biological activity. In addition, gene multiplication may lead to increased expression of a particular enzyme in certain individuals. This leads to the "very extensive metaboliser phenotype" (Mulder, 2006). Interindividual differences in drug metabolism can therefore be influenced by molecular genetic and gene expression differences in drug-metabolizing systems. This variation in metabolism of xenobiotics is not represented by normal clinical signs or biochemical tests. It manifests itself only when the patient is exposed to the medication.

10.12 INVESTIGATION OF PHARMACOKINETICS IN SPECIAL POPULATIONS

Once a drug is approved for marketing, it would be preferable if a single dosing regimen could be used for the vast majority of patients. However, there are many potential sources of variation in how individuals, and identifiable subgroups, react to a given drug. These include:

- Genetic differences. Patients show a wide variation in both the extent of liver biotransformation and the range of metabolic pathways used to eliminate drugs. Differences in the metabolism of the drug can lead to a smaller clinical effect than desired, a greater clinical effect than desired (e.g., an antihypertensive causing hypotension), or a more toxic effect than desired.
- Gender.
- Ethnicity.
- Health condition and nutritional status.
- Previous and ongoing exposure to other drugs.
- Renal or hepatic impairment.
- Age.

The inclusion and exclusion criteria that are used in clinical trials can be extensive, and they usually mean that the subject population in a trial is relatively homogenous. For example, potential subjects who have other illnesses or medical conditions are typically excluded. This includes hepatic and renal impairment. Clinical efficacy trials typically exclude subjects with renal or hepatic impairment in order to study how the drug performs in nonimpaired individuals. This strategy is useful for reducing variability of drug response in the trial and facilitating the best possible evaluation of the "pure" treatment effect in the "average" person. However, practicing clinicians do not treat a stream of average patients: A clinician's patients are not likely to be homogenous (see Chapter 13). Therefore, the drug's safety and efficacy in special populations need to be investigated in due course, particularly if the drug's target population is likely to include many such patients. In addition to individuals with hepatic or renal impairment, it is also of interest to examine responses to the drug in the elderly.

This brings up a general point of particular relevance in extrapolating the results of clinical trials to a larger population of patients. To apply evidence that was the result of a statistical inference in a certain population to a different population is a clinical inference (see Katz, 2001, as cited in Section 13.7.1). Making this leap is the product of sound clinical judgment and the weighing of benefits and risks for a particular patient. Such clinical practice is expected—it is one of many responsibilities shouldered by clinicians—and this is one of the primary reasons for the postmarketing surveillance discussed in Chapter 13.

10.12.1 Hepatic Impairment

The liver plays a central role in the absorption and disposition kinetics of most drugs. The majority of drug metabolism takes place in the liver, with some metabolism occurring in the kidneys and lungs. The liver is a large organ that can lose a significant percentage of its mass while retaining its metabolic function.

Biochemical indicators show only cell damage, not the amount of mass remaining. They provide only limited amounts of information about the ability of the liver to metabolize xenobiotic compounds such as drugs.

There are many forms of liver disease and these appear to differ in their effects on drug clearance. Additionally, age, genetics, and drug interactions can produce huge variability in liver enzyme function, as can comorbidities such as cardiac function, thyroid status, diabetes, and alcohol intake. The first-pass effect, while useful for protecting the rest of the body from toxic effects of xenobiotics, can be harmful to the liver. It can lead to high uptake (exposure) and high bioactivation activity in the liver, leading to hepatotoxicity.

There are no clear markers of liver dysfunction. Standard liver function tests such as rises in alkaline phosphatase and alanine aminotransferase (see Section 11.10.1) are only crude markers of liver function and have not proved useful in characterizing liver function in relation to drug pharmacokinetics. The effect of liver dysfunction on drug clearance is therefore often addressed descriptively rather than quantitatively (see Weeks and Tomlin, 2006, for further discussion).

10.12.2 Renal Insufficiency

While renal contribution to overall metabolism is less than hepatic contribution, renal metabolism is of clinical importance. The kidney, in particular the renal cortex, contains many of the same metabolic enzymes found in the liver, including CYPs. Serum creatinine and creatinine clearance are the typical methods used to assess renal function, although 24-hour urine collection can also be used. These are reliable indicators of renal clearance.

Renal insufficiency has a profound effect on the disposition and handling of drugs by the body. Reduced renal excretion is not the only change in drug disposition in patients with renal insufficiency. There are also changes in oral bioavailability, protein and tissue binding, distribution, and even hepatic metabolism. Drugs that are excreted by the kidneys in their active form or as active metabolites are eliminated at a reduced rate, which causes accumulation of drug, which can lead to adverse effects. Clinical care of patients with renal insufficiency therefore needs special attention (see Ashley, 2006, for further discussion).

10.12.3 The Elderly

The elderly represent a growing proportion of the total population, and it is necessary to appreciate the age-associated physiological changes that occur in these patients and their effects on the disposition of drugs.

Metabolic capacity changes across the life span. Hepatic metabolic capacity rises to a peak around 16 years of age and then declines. In the elderly, hepatic blood flow is reduced by up to 40%. This means that delivery of the drug to the liver is less, leading to reduced metabolism and a longer half-life. Elimination of drug and also drug metabolites is affected. Renal mass may decrease with age, as may renal functioning. The presence of concurrent disease can also play a role here. Hypertension or diabetes may affect renal sufficiency independently of age.

In general, older patients handle many drugs differently from younger adult patients. While there are differences among drug classes, the usual consequence is increased toxicity (see Cairns, 2006, for further discussion).

10.12.4 Pediatric Populations

Various regulatory agencies around the world are working to increase the number of clinical trials involving children. The FDA's Office of Pediatric Therapeutics focuses on both clinical and ethical aspects of clinical research in pediatric populations and works to increase the scientific understanding of the medical needs of children.

Physiological processes that influence pharmacokinetic variables in the infant change significantly in the first years of life, particularly during the first few months (Koren, 2004). Metabolism is quite different in early neonatal life than later, with different enzymatic systems approaching adult characteristics at different rates. Generally, enzymes may be poorly developed at birth, and specific metabolic pathways may be absent. Enzyme maturation is complete about 6–8 months of age. As with elderly patients, the neonate's decreased ability to metabolize drugs means that many drugs have slow clearance rates and prolonged elimination half-lives. If drug doses and dosing schedules are not altered appropriately, the neonate is predisposed to adverse effects. Additionally, the process of maturation must be considered when chronic administration of drugs is necessary in young patients.

Because of differences in pharmacokinetics in infants and children, it may not be appropriate simply to proportionately reduce the adult dose. If it is available, the most reliable pediatric dose information available is usually the information provided by the manufacturer in the package insert: however, this information is not available for the majority of products (Koren, 2004). Recently, the FDA has moved toward more explicit expectations that sponsors conduct appropriate clinical evaluations of new products in infants and children. (See also http://www.fda.gov/cder/pediatric/Summaryreview.htm).

The issue of pediatric drug evaluation is considered again in Section 14.10 when discussing the FDA's March 2006 Critical Path Opportunities List: Pediatrics is the sixth item on this list.

10.13 TYPES OF SAFETY-RELATED DATA

Safety-related data can be considered at three levels:

- The extent of exposure.
- Common adverse events and serious adverse events and other significant adverse events.
- Common laboratory tests.

10.13.1 Extent of Exposure

The extent of subjects' exposure to a drug during a clinical trial is a determinant of the extent to which safety can be assessed from the data collected. Extent of exposure can be characterized in several ways:

- Number of subjects exposed.
- Duration of exposure.
- Dose(s) to which subjects were exposed.
- Definition of daily dose levels: maximum dose for each subject, dose with the longest exposure for each subject, mean daily dose, cumulative dose.
- Numbers of subjects exposed to the dose(s) for certain periods of time.
- Profile of exposure for different subject populations: subjects broken down by age, gender, ethnic subgroup, disease severity, concurrent illnesses.
- Combined dose-duration: numbers of subjects exposed for a given duration to the most common dose or highest recommended dose.

10.13.2 Adverse Events

The varying nomenclature used to describe safety data in clinical trials can be confusing. Some of the terms used are:

- Adverse events.
- Adverse experiences.
- Adverse drug reactions.
- Side effects.
- Severe adverse events.
- Significant adverse events.
- Serious adverse events (SAEs).
- Treatment-emergent adverse events.
- Risks.
- Toxicities.

ICH E6 (R1) provides the following definition of adverse event:

> Any untoward medical occurrence in a patient or clinical investigation subject administered a pharmaceutical product and which does not necessarily have a causal relationship with the treatment. An adverse event (AE) can therefore be any unfavourable and unintended sign (including an abnormal laboratory finding), symptom, or disease temporally associated with the use of a medicinal (investigational) product, whether or not associated with the medicinal (investigational) product (p. 2).

ICH E2A provides a definition of adverse drug reaction that is applicable during preapproval clinical experiences with a new medicinal product:

> All noxious and unintended responses to a medicinal product related to any dose should be considered adverse drug reactions.

The phrase "responses to a medicinal product" in this definition means that a causal relationship between a medicinal product and an adverse event is at least a reasonable possibility, i.e., "the relationship cannot be ruled out."

When reporting the results of a clinical trial, it is of interest to know about the frequency of all adverse events that occurred in a trial and any relationships with time, demographic characteristics, and relation to drug dose or concentration. It is also of interest to differentiate as much as possible between those adverse events that are drug related, i.e., those where there is a "reasonable possibility" of a relationship to the drug administered, and those that are not. There are various ways to do this, including listings and in-text summary tables. Listings are comprehensive lists that provide all information concerning adverse events. Listings are appended to a clinical study report that is submitted to a regulatory agency. In-text summary tables are placed in the body of the text in clinical study reports. These in-text tables summarize the number of subjects in each treatment group in whom the event occurred and the rate of occurrence. Sometimes, a sponsor will report adverse events that occurred in at least a given percentage of the subjects in either group (information for both treatment groups is presented in each case).

When adverse drug reactions occur that may be significant enough to lead to important changes in the way the medicinal product is developed, these should be reported promptly to regulatory agencies. This applies particularly to reactions which, in their most severe forms, threaten life or function (ICH E2A). These reactions are deemed serious.

It is important to differentiate in this context between the terms "serious" and "severe." As ICH E2A notes, the term severe is typically used to describe the intensity or severity of a specific event: mild, moderate, and severe are typical categories used for describing degrees of severity. It is noteworthy that a severe event, e.g., a severe headache, may be "of relatively minor medical significance" (ICH E2A). It is seriousness, not severity, that serves as the guide for reporting obligations to regulatory agencies.

Accordingly, ICH E2A provides the following definition of a serious event:

> A serious adverse event (experience) or reaction is any untoward medical occurrence that at any dose:
>
> - Results in death,
> - Is life threatening (NOTE: The term "life-threatening" in the definition of "serious" refers to an event in which the patient was at risk of death

at the time of the event; it does not refer to an event which hypothetically might have caused death if it were more severe.),
- Requires inpatient hospitalization or prolongation of existing hospitalization,
- Results in persistent or significant disability/incapacity, or
- Is a congenital anomaly/birth defect (p. 3).

10.14 Acquisition of Safety Data

During the course of a clinical trial it is likely that most subjects will have some form of adverse events (AEs). The longer the study and the sicker the subjects are, the more AEs there will be. Since AEs do not actually have to be related to the treatment, the sites report "everything from colds, to falls, to car accidents, to murder, as well as all the typical medical conditions that might be monitored by any doctor" (Prokscha, 2007). Adverse events can be grouped into various categories. Two of these are:

- Open AE reports. The open form is the most common. The nature of the AE is recorded in the subject's own words or in the investigator's version of the subject's words.
- Expected signs and symptoms. When a treatment has already shown a history of certain kinds of AEs, there may be particular interest in the frequency and severity of these specific AEs during the course of the study: The term AEs of special interest is sometimes used in this context. A list of these signs/symptoms is provided, and both subjects and investigators look for these events, identifying those that occurred with a yes/no answer.

In both cases, the investigator generally makes an assessment of:

- Severity.
- Relationship to the treatment.
- Action taken.
- Start and stop dates or whether the event is ongoing.

10.14.1 Management of Adverse Event Data

The management of safety data requires not only all the care that management of every other type of data collected requires (recall Section 5.9) but also some extra considerations. The first of these is the process of coding. To facilitate the summarization of AE data that are collected in the subjects' own words (or the investigators' version of their words), and can therefore be heterogeneous, a degree of uniformity has to be introduced. For example, the terms "headache," "mild headache," and "aching head" should all be counted as the same kind of event (Prokscha, 2007). The same concept applies to medications: Tylenol and acetaminophen should be classified as the same drug.

The process of classifying the reported terms by using a large list of possibilities is known as coding. This is done by matching, or coding, each reported AE against a dictionary (given the sheer volume of safety data, this process is typically done via computerized "autocoding"). A widely used dictionary is MedDRA, the *Medical Dictionary for Regulatory Activities*. This dictionary is particularly comprehensive in that it includes terms used in various contexts, including:

- Diseases.
- Diagnoses.
- Signs.
- Symptoms.
- Therapeutic indications.

One notable difficulty that occurs in the coding process is splitting terms when the initial report contains two terms, e.g., "headache and nausea." Simply splitting this into two terms is problematic, since "it is not clear whether all the data associated with each term (onset date, severity, etc) apply equally to both terms" (Prokscha, 2007). As the FDA becomes more vigilant regarding safety data, companies are becoming more conservative in handling safety data. The current trend is for data management to issue queries to the sites for all discrepancies or problems associated with AE data, including splitting terms (Prokscha, 2007).

10.14.2 Management of Serious Adverse Event Data

Serious adverse events that are seen in clinical trials and in the general use of marketed products need to be reported directly to a safety group or safety coordinator. Safety groups tend to operate and maintain their own databases for these SAE reports, or cases, because of the detailed information related to each case that they must collect (Prokscha, 2007). Each SAE case is initially entered in this system and then updated as follow-up information becomes available.

In addition to the system of recording that has just been described, SAEs that occur during clinical trials are also recorded on the case report forms along with all other data collected in the trial. This version of the SAE information is then entered into the clinical data management system, which is the source of SAE data used in the trial analyses that are reported to regulatory agencies. The existence of two databases causes additional care to be taken with SAE data. Before the end of a clinical trial, the SAE data in the safety group's system must be compared with the SAE data in the clinical data management system to ensure that all SAEs were collected and reported properly in both systems. This process is called reconciliation (Prokscha, 2007).

10.15 COMMON LABORATORY TESTS

Like analysis plans for AEs (see Section 10.17.2), analysis plans for laboratory data can also be relatively vague. One common approach here is to examine the change from baseline to the last treatment visit. There are several ways that "change" can be defined and quantified. One method is to calculate the absolute change. When using absolute changes, the data used in the analysis are continuous data, and methods such as the *t*-test can be used in the analysis. A second approach is to consider the number of subjects in each treatment group whose measurements were outside the "normal range" at baseline and at the last treatment visit (the normal range must be defined in the study protocol). The second approach produces frequency data, which means that different analytical strategies are needed (see Chow and Liu, 2004, for further discussion).

10.15.1 Clinical Chemistry Data

There is a very wide range of clinical chemistry tests that can be conducted. For example:

Liver function tests:
- ALP (alkaline phosphatase).
- ALT/SGPT (serum glutamic pyruvate transaminase).
- AST/SGOT (serum glutamic oxaloacetin transaminase).
- Albumin.
- Bilirubin.
- Globulin.
- LDH (lactic acid dehydrogenase).
- Total protein.

Renal function tests:
- BUN (blood-urea-nitrogen).
- Creatinine.
- Creatinine clearance.

10.15.2 Central Laboratories

Most therapeutic confirmatory trials are run at multiple investigative sites in order to enroll enough subjects. Central laboratories are testing laboratories to which samples from all of the investigative sites in a clinical trial are shipped. This strategy has two important advantages compared with using a large collection of "local laboratories," laboratories close to each investigative site:

- Assurance that the laboratory conducting the analyses of the samples is compliant with cGCP is much easier.
- Statistical difficulties associated with analyzing "pooled laboratory data" are avoided.

It is ultimately the sponsor's responsibility to ensure that cGCP is followed in its clinical trials, even though some of the work is contracted out to CROs and other service providers. With regard to analytical laboratories, GCP guidances require that all laboratories have full documentation, data-audit trails, standard procedures, trained staff, archives of samples and data, and routine quality assurance inspections (Prokscha, 2007). If multiple laboratories were to be used, the sponsor would need assurance that GCP requirements were met for every one. In contrast, if a central laboratory is used and all samples are shipped to it, the sponsor only needs to check GCP compliance at that laboratory.

With regard to the second advantage of central laboratories, analysis of data that have been collected from many sources and then "pooled" into one data set can lead to considerable statistical problems. Since the majority of laboratory measurements are surrogates and reference ranges can vary from analytical method to method, many different types of errors can occur during laboratory testing. These can be due to variation in many aspects of data collection, including the technician, an instrument, the environment, and the reagents used. Therefore, statistical analyses using data that are pooled from many different local laboratories can be problematic. While statistical approaches to standardize values from several local laboratories, each with their own reference ranges, have been described (Chuang-Stein, 1992), central laboratories provide a real statistical advantage in this context. All samples are analyzed in the same manner in the same laboratory, thereby providing a much better data set. As Chow and Liu (2004) noted, "laboratory data obtained from central laboratories are more accurate and reliable compared with those obtained from local laboratories."

It should be noted that using central laboratories can be considerably more expensive than would be the case if samples were sent to local laboratories close to each investigational site. The central laboratory used can be many miles from some of the investigational sites, even in another country or continent. Expedited shipping under very carefully controlled conditions is necessary to ensure that the samples arrive at the central laboratory quickly and safely. However, obtaining optimum quality laboratory data is critical, and the necessary expenditure involved here is well worthwhile.

10.16 ANALYSIS POPULATIONS USED FOR SAFETY DATA

Various analysis populations for clinical trial data can be defined and used in statistical analyses. Of relevance in this chapter are the intent-to-treat (ITT) population and the safety population (additional populations are considered in the following chapter). The ITT population comprises all subjects in a clinical trial that were randomized to a treatment group, regardless if any data were actually collected from them. The safety population is a specified subset of the ITT population and is defined as the population of subjects who received at least one dose of a treatment (only subjects who took a drug are at risk for an adverse event caused by the drug). Both the ITT and the safety populations can be used in the analysis of safety data.

10.17 PRESENTATION OF DATA IN REGULATORY CLINICAL STUDY REPORTS

As noted in Section 10.1, in addition to discussing safety assessment in clinical trials, this chapter provides an overview of clinical trials in general. As well as reviewing different types of trials in Section 10.2, this section provides a brief introduction to presenting general clinical trial data in clinical study reports before looking specifically at the presentation of safety data.

10.17.1 Study Population Results

Describing, or summarizing, the tremendous amount of data that are collected in a clinical trial is typically a very useful first step in reporting the results of the trial. Simple descriptors such as the total number of participants in the trial, the numbers that received the drug treatment and the placebo treatment, respectively, and the average age of the participants in each treatment group help to set the scene for more detailed reporting.

The Study Population Results section often comes at the beginning of the Results section in the clinical study report and tells the reviewer about the disposition of the subjects in the study. The ITT population is typically used for these descriptions. Much of the information may be presented in tabular form in in-text tables to make the regulatory reviewers' task as easy as possible. All data that are reported in a clinical study report need to be verifiable against original source tables provided in the overall submission, and so each in-text table indicates where the source data relevant to the entries in the table are located.

Table 10.2 provides an example of an in-text table that summarizes subject accountability. This in-text table of hypothetical data is identified by the title associated with it, and the information in the headers provides more detail concerning the nature of the data presented. In this example, clinical trial ABC was conducted using a drug treatment group and a placebo treatment group, and data for the ITT population are presented.

Table 10.2. Subject Accountability (ITT Population: Study ABC)

	Number (%) of Subjects	
	Drug (*N*=200)	Placebo (*N*=200)
Completion Status		
Completed study	160 (80)	180 (90)
Withdrew prematurely	40 (20)	20 (10)
Reasons for Premature Withdrawal		
Adverse event	20 (10)	6 (3)
Withdrew consent	10 (5)	4 (2)
Protocol violation	10 (5)	8 (4)
Other	0	2 (1)

Several comments about these hypothetical data are appropriate. It is possible but unlikely that the numbers of subjects for the two treatment groups would be identical in a real study. Ideally, they would be fairly close, since, as noted in Section 5.6.2, equal numbers provide the most powerful test of differences between two groups. Since the number of subjects in each group would likely be different, presenting percentages as well as absolute numbers is useful, since the percentages allow for differing totals of subjects in each group. Third, the numbers of subjects in the individual categories must add up to the respective group totals. Fourth, explanation of the "other" reasons for premature withdrawal may be useful and could be presented in text form above or below the table or in footnote form immediately underneath the table.

It is worth noting here that documentation of premature withdrawals from a study is important for various reasons. The implications of premature withdrawals are different in the analysis of safety and the analysis of efficacy. From a safety perspective, these data relate to tolerability of the drug. From an efficacy perspective, dropouts lead to missing data, and the way(s) that missing data are addressed is important from the point of view of full interpretation of the analysis presented. The issue of missing data is addressed in Section 11.2.4.

A similar table may be presented for demographic characteristics. Specific characteristics that are important can vary from study to study, but typical ones include gender, age, race, and baseline data of relevance, e.g., weight, blood pressure, and heart rate. Information concerning the use of concomitant or concurrent medications and evaluations of subject adherence or compliance with the trial's treatment schedule is also typically presented.

10.17.2 Presentation of Safety Data

Safety data are predominantly presented in a descriptive manner at this time, but it is likely that analytical strategies will be increasingly used.

Descriptive approaches to safety data.

Given the interest in reducing potential toxicity at the drug discovery and design stage (discussed in Chapter 3), the emphasis on safety in nonclinical research (discussed in Chapter 4), and the extensive safety monitoring in early phase clinical trials, it may come as somewhat of a surprise that methodology for the analysis of safety data in therapeutic clinical trials is not rigorously defined. Chow and Liu (2004) commented on the problems in defining, capturing, and evaluating safety-related data and also noted that both FDA and ICH guidelines state that every adverse event need not be subjected to rigorous statistical evaluation. As a result, "the analysis of adverse events is basically descriptive in nature" (Chow and Liu, 2004). Descriptive statistics for adverse events obtained from clinical trials typically include rates of occurrence of adverse events in exposed groups overall and among groups of subjects (e.g., according to age and gender) to look for any potential patterns of differential rates of adverse events.

Comparing rates of adverse events between two groups may seem a straightforward and reasonable strategy. However, such a comparison is only reasonable if the length of observation (i.e., "time at risk") is equal between the groups. O'Neill (1987) has proposed alternative methods of presenting adverse event data that take into account varying times at risk. These alternative approaches can shed light on the time course of the adverse events.

One of two possible populations is usually chosen for use in the presentation of safety data. Chow and Liu (2004) suggested that all subjects entered into treatment who receive as little as one dose of the treatment should be included in the safety analysis, and if not, a reason should be provided. This population is called the safety population. The ITT population can also be used for safety analyses.

Several summary tables are commonly presented to report safety data. Two examples of typical formats are provided here. Table 10.3 shows the format for the overall summary of adverse events falling within several adverse event categories. Such "table shells" are typically prepared by medical writers in advance of the study results being available and are based on the clinical study protocol and/or the statistical analysis plan written before the study started. Preparation in advance of the availability of the data saves time during the preparation of the clinical study report once the data are available.

Table 10.3. Overall Summary of AEs (Safety Population: Study ABC)

Adverse Events	Number (%) of Subjects	
	Drug (*N*=200)	Placebo (*N*=200)
Pretreatment AEs	xx (xx)	xx (xx)
Treatment AEs	xx (xx)	xx (xx)
Drug-related AEs	xx (xx)	xx (xx)
SAEs	xx (xx)	xx (xx)
AEs leading to withdrawal	xx (xx)	xx (xx)

Table 10.4 shows the format for the summary of the most common adverse events. The meaning of the phrase "most common" must be defined every time it is used. In this example it is defined by the statement "Greater or equal to 10%." Note that it is possible (indeed very likely) that the incidence of side effects will not be identical in the two treatment groups. Some adverse events that occur in ≥10% in the drug treatment group may occur in less than 10% in the placebo treatment group, and vice versa. Data for both treatment groups employed will be provided for any adverse event listed for either group. Data are often presented in descending order of occurrence. Similar presentations of these data are included in package inserts for marketed products. While not specifically discussed in this book, package inserts can reasonably be considered as the driving force behind clinical trials and the culmination of their activities.

Table 10.4. Most Common (≥10% in Either Treatment Group) Adverse Events (Safety Population: Study ABC)

	Number (%) of Subjects	
	Drug (*N*=200)	Placebo (*N*=200)
Any event	xx (xx)	xx (xx)
Headache	xx (xx)	xx (xx)
Nausea	xx (xx)	xx (xx)
Insomnia	xx (xx)	xx (xx)
Fatigue	xx (xx)	xx (xx)
Dizziness	xx (xx)	xx (xx)
Etc.	xx (xx)	xx (xx)

Analytical approaches to safety data.

The analytical approach to safety data is limited but growing (Dubey et al., 2006). Some suitable statistical techniques that can be employed include Fisher's exact test, the Mantel-Haenszel test, and the adapted Cochran-Mantel-Haenszel test, all of which can be used to compare adverse event rates between treatment groups (see Chow and Liu, 2004, for further details).

Analytical approaches to safety data are very different from the analytical approaches to efficacy data that are discussed in the next chapter. Some of the reasons for these differences are:

- Safety analyses are not typically prespecified in the study protocol and/or the study analysis plan. Studies are typically powered on efficacy outcomes (the primary objective in therapeutic confirmatory trials: see Chapter 9), and the sample size that results from this sample-size estimation may be considerably smaller than would be needed for a thorough investigation of safety data.
- They involve numerous outcome events (e.g., all sorts of adverse events, laboratory tests, ECG tests). This means that considerable attention must be paid to issues of multiplicity (see Section 7.10), making it important to protect Type I error. A "significant" result is therefore difficult to interpret.
- Once all of the necessary multiplicity considerations have been implemented, most studies are not sufficiently large to achieve statistical significance when comparing incidence rates of safety variables between treatment groups. Therefore, safety analyses may be regarded as hypothesis generating more so than hypothesis testing.

One approach that can be adopted in the analysis of safety data is to identify a finding of interest and then look across different trials for consistency. In the case of safety data evaluation, this may be more informative than the magnitude of specific p-values obtained. Confidence intervals of adverse rates can be informative (particularly when they are narrow) and may be useful to regulatory agencies in their decision making (Dubey et al., 2006).

11

Efficacy Assessment in Clinical Trials

11.1 Introduction

In addition to having an acceptable safety profile, an investigational drug needs to display beneficial therapeutic effects. This takes us into the realm of therapeutic exploratory and therapeutic confirmatory trials. The statistical approaches discussed in this chapter are characteristic of those employed in these trials.

The previous chapter discussed the (currently) relatively loosely defined statistical approaches to safety data collected in clinical trials. In contrast, there are widely accepted statistical methods for demonstrating efficacy in clinical trials. As has been noted several times in this book, if the study design and methodology have been appropriate and have led to the collection of optimum quality data, the statistical analysis and interpretation of efficacy data are relatively straightforward. The clinical (biological) interpretation of efficacy data is typically not quite as clear-cut, but there are widely accepted methodologies that are very useful in this realm too. Of particular importance here is the expert judgment of the clinicians who will review the statistical results with the statisticians and the rest of the study team.

11.1.1 Superiority, Equivalence, Noninferiority, and Bioequivalence Trials

In previous chapters, discussion has focused on superiority trials. These trials are conducted to demonstrate to the satisfaction of regulatory agencies that the investigational drug is "superior" in efficacy to a placebo, or possibly superior in efficacy to an active comparator. In addition, this chapter also introduces other study designs that are very informative and, in some cases, necessary.

Equivalence trials are conducted to demonstrate therapeutic equivalence with an active comparator drug, which is often the current "gold standard" treatment (see Section 12.3.1 for discussion of gold standard therapy). The intent is to provide compelling evidence that the efficacy of the investigational drug is "equivalent" to that of the active comparator drug. This type of trial is typically conducted if it is believed that the new drug has benefits such as a better safety profile. The statistical definition of equivalent is addressed in this chapter. Noninferiority trials are similar to equivalence trials, but they take the concept a little further. The investigational drug may have a safety profile that is so much better than the safety profile of the active comparator that clinicians are prepared to accept slightly less efficacy. The definition of slightly less is couched in terms of the new drug being "noninferior." The statistical definition of noninferiority is addressed here.

Bioequivalence trials are typically conducted to demonstrate that a new formulation of a drug has equivalent characteristics to an existing formulation

New Drug Development: Design, Methodology, and Analysis. By J. Rick Turner

of the drug and to investigate whether a different way of administering the drug is preferable or a good alternative in certain situations when the original method of administration is not feasible. In this study design, both efficacy and safety characteristics are considered.

11.1.2 Group Sequential and Adaptive Study Designs

The study design that we have focused on so far can be called a fixed design or a fixed sample design, one in which there is no latitude to deviate from the precise plans detailed in the study protocol and the statistical analysis plan. The study design is specified at the beginning of the trial, the number of subjects that will be enrolled is clearly stated, and the plan for data analysis is laid out in detail before the study starts. Once the trial has commenced, it progresses as planned until its conclusion, at which time the statistical analyses are conducted. In contrast, group sequential designs and adaptive designs have inherent flexibility to "change" in midstream. It must be emphasized here that, while the precise nature of any change that may occur is not known at the outset, precise rules that determine the permissibility of any changes must be specified in detail in the study protocol.

Both group sequential and adaptive designs incorporate interim analyses. Interim analyses are analyses that are done during an ongoing clinical trial. Their purpose is different in each of these designs. In group sequential trials, the purpose of interim analyses is to determine if the trial should be terminated at that point for one of several reasons, including evidence that already demonstrates in a compelling manner that the drug is effective or that it is toxic. In adaptive trials, the purpose of interim analyses is to determine how best to modify the remainder of the trial in order to increase the amount of useful information that can be gained from the trial.

11.2 ANALYSIS POPULATIONS FOR EFFICACY ANALYSES

The ITT analysis population and the per-protocol (efficacy or evaluable) population are typically used in efficacy analyses. As described in the previous chapter, the ITT population comprises all subjects in a clinical trial that were randomized to a treatment group, regardless if any data were actually collected from them.

11.2.1 The Intent-to-Treat Population

In many clinical trials, especially trials that occur later in a new drug development program, analyses are first conducted on the ITT population. These analyses are considered to be the primary analyses. Intent-to-treat analysis provides a conservative strategy in the sense that it tends to bias against finding the results that the researcher "hopes" for (recall the discussion in Section 7.2.1 regarding hope). The ITT population therefore comprises the "purest" population of subjects in the trial and therefore the most appropriate population from which to make inferences to any larger population outside the parameters of the specific trial.

When attempting to demonstrate the efficacy of a new drug, the use of data that do not favor this desired outcome is deemed appropriate. Then, if there is compelling evidence of the drug's efficacy, this evidence will be particularly noteworthy. This is the case for the ITT population. Analysis of the ITT population data may also provide estimates of treatment effects that are more likely to mirror those observed in subsequent clinical practice, i.e., the treatment of patients in real-world settings, should the drug subsequently be approved for marketing.

11.2.2 The Per-Protocol Population

The Per-protocol population is comprised of subjects whose participation and involvement in the trial was compliant with all of the requirements and activities detailed in the study protocol. The per-protocol population is a specified subset of the ITT population: Subjects who are not compliant are excluded from the per-protocol data set. It should be noted that it is not simply subjects themselves that cause deviations from the protocol: An investigator can also be responsible for not conducting parts of the trial appropriately. It was noted in Section 5.7.2 that excessively long study protocols can be associated with lack of compliance on the part of the investigators. Exclusion of subjects whose activities violated the protocol because the investigator did not conduct part of the trial properly is a very real outcome of this problem.

In contrast to the conservative ITT analysis, analysis of the per-protocol population may maximize the opportunity to demonstrate efficacy: the per-protocol population is the population in which the treatment is likely to perform best. Adherence to the protocol may be related to the treatment and outcome (Kay, 2005). This is why the per-protocol analysis is considered secondary to the more conservative ITT analysis.

11.2.3 Using Both Analysis Populations

As far as regulatory authorities are concerned, it is encouraging if the results from the ITT efficacy analysis and the per-protocol efficacy analysis are qualitatively similar. The word "qualitative" in the last sentence may seem a strange one in a book that focuses on quantitative statements and quantitative analyses. However, it provides another illustration that the skillful practice of Statistics is both a science and an art. Strict adherence to statistical rules and computational accuracy are certainly fundamental requirements in obtaining the results from statistical analyses, but, as well as interpreting the results of individual analyses, skilled and experienced statisticians are also able to look at data in a more global manner and use their expertise to make more global interpretations.

If the picture painted by both the ITT analysis and the per-protocol analysis is similar, overall confidence in the trial results is increased. However, if they are not similar, questions may be raised as to why they are not. Relatedly, if the per-protocol population is a lot smaller than the ITT population (it will almost certainly be somewhat smaller), regulatory reviewers will wonder why. Were there a lot of major protocol violations? Were a lot of subjects removed for the same protocol violation? Were many of the subjects with protocol violations enrolled at the same investigative site? Are there any systematic problems in the conduct of the trial? These issues can all reduce overall confidence in the trial's findings.

11.2.4 Missing Data

It was noted in Section 10.17.1 that, in efficacy assessment, the way(s) that missing data are addressed is important from the point of view of full interpretation of the analysis presented. As Piantadosi (2005) noted, there are only three generic analytic approaches to coping with missing values:

- Disregard the observations that contain a missing value.
- Disregard a particular variable if it has a high frequency of missing values.
- Replace the missing values by some appropriate value.

The last of these approaches is called imputation of missing values. As Piantadosi (2005) commented, while this approach sounds a lot like "making up data," when done properly it may be the most sensible strategy. While techniques for addressing missing data can be technically difficult, one commonly used, simple imputation method is called last observation carried forward (LOCF). In a study with repeated measurements over time, the most recent observation replaces any subsequent missing observations (Piantadosi, 2005, see also Molenberghs and Kenward, 2007).

11.3 HYPOTHESIS TESTING IS INTEGRAL TO ALL OF THE DESIGNS DISCUSSED HERE

While the practical details of the statistical approaches employed in equivalence, noninferiority, and bioequivalence trials are different from those employed in superiority trials, all of the approaches employ hypothesis testing. The differences lie in the nature of the hypotheses that are created and then tested.

Discussions in Chapter 7 explained how hypothesis testing is structured in superiority trials. A null hypothesis is established that states that there is no statistically significant difference between the investigational drug's efficacy and the control's efficacy. In slightly imprecise terms (but the concept is important here), the null hypothesis states that the test drug and the comparator drug have similar efficacy. The statistical methodology used in superiority trials looks for compelling evidence to reject the null hypothesis.

In the case of equivalence, noninferiority, and bioequivalence trials, the null hypotheses established are different from the null hypothesis established in superiority trials. In addition, the null hypothesis in each case is unique, and hence they all differ from each other. However, they share a basic similarity. The null hypothesis for each of these designs states, in effect, that the test drug and the comparator drug do not have similar efficacy. As in all hypothesis testing, the statistical methodologies used look for compelling evidence to reject the respective null hypothesis in each case.

It is noteworthy that, while the null hypothesis in each of the trial designs discussed (superiority, equivalence, noninferiority, and equivalence) is different, the hypothesis testing approach in each case is fundamentally similar to that in every other case. In each instance it is "hoped" that the null hypothesis will be rejected in favor of the research hypothesis.

11.4 SUPERIORITY TRIALS

Two common statistical techniques that are typically used to analyze efficacy data in superiority trials are *t*-tests and ANOVA. In parallel group trials, the independent groups *t*-test and the independent groups ANOVA discussed in Chapter 7 would be used. Another important aspect of the statistical methodology employed in superiority trials, the use of CIs (confidence intervals) to estimate the clinical significance of a treatment effect, was discussed in Chapter 8. These discussions are not repeated here. Instead, some additional aspects of statistical methodology that are relevant to superiority trials are discussed.

11.4.1 Well-Defined Study Objectives and Endpoints

All of the studies that are performed before a therapeutic confirmatory trial is started collect information that facilitates a logical scientific progression from FTIH studies to the point where the therapeutic confirmatory trial is appropriate. In a real sense, all of these studies, and all of the information gained to date, have had one purpose: to allow the primary objective in the therapeutic confirmatory trial to be stated as simply as possible. In this context, the word "simple" is not pejorative. To the contrary, a primary objective that can be stated simply can be tested simply, i.e., in a straightforward and unambiguous manner. This is a highly desirable attribute in a primary objective.

The number of objectives that should be incorporated in any clinical trial is often a topic of considerable debate among study teams. One argument often propounded is that, while taking all the trouble to conduct the trial, why not collect as much data as possible and ask as many questions as possible? This approach leads to a large number of study objectives, sometimes broken down into primary objectives, secondary objectives, and even tertiary objectives. Proponents of this approach see it as commendable to have all of these objectives specified *a priori*, since this removes the possibility of any later intimation that these topics of interest arose after the data were analyzed. However, this approach leads to serious statistical problems, and it can compromise the weight of any particular piece of evidence that is presented to regulatory agencies.

Section 7.10 discussed the concerns that accompany multiple comparisons and multiplicity. As noted there, when adopting the 5% significance level (α =0.05) it is likely that, when 20 separate comparisons are made, a Type I error will occur. That is, a statistically significant result will be "found" by chance alone. The greater the number of objectives presented in a study protocol, the greater the number of comparisons that will be made at the analysis stage, and the greater the chance of a Type I error. As Machin and Campbell (2005) commented, "If there are too many endpoints defined, the multiplicity of comparisons then made at the analysis stage may result in spurious statistical significance."

By the time a therapeutic confirmatory trial is appropriate, it should be possible to state a single primary objective (or perhaps two if the sponsor really feels that this is appropriate) that is clinically relevant and biologically plausible. One primary objective also means that sample-size estimation can be based on that objective and the associated estimated treatment effect of interest (recall the discussions in Chapter 9).

These comments do not minimize the difficulty of choosing just one or two primary objectives. It is legitimate in some studies to be interested in more than one endpoint and also to be interested in additional aspects such as quality-of life (QoL) scores. Quality of life is an extremely important consideration and one that is of particular relevance to long-term pharmacological therapy. Even if a disease or condition cannot be cured, keeping the symptomology at levels acceptable to a patient can be a tremendous success. However, from a statistical point of view, assessing quality of life in clinical trials involves taking many measures, and if these are analyzed separately, the multiplicity problem is of real concern. Machin and Campbell (2005) suggested that, in cases where additional evaluations are included in addition to the primary (more clinical) endpoints, study design should focus on the few key endpoints. In turn, at the analysis stage, these endpoints provide the focus for rigorous statistical analysis and interpretation. Any secondary endpoints included in the study protocol might be summarized and less formal statistical comparisons made for them.

11.4.2 Analysis of Covariance

While the process of randomization is very efficient in distributing random sources of variation among treatment groups, it is certainly possible (and indeed likely) that the drug treatment group and the control treatment group will differ to some extent in some ways. For example, it is unlikely that subjects' weights will be identical, and it is therefore unlikely that the mean weights of the treatment groups will be the same. It was noted in Section 4.5.1 that, in nonclinical studies, the technique of censored randomization is used to make the weights of the animals in the two treatment groups as similar as the researcher wishes them to be. This strategy is not feasible in clinical trials, but a statistical technique called analysis of covariance (ANCOVA) permits differences in other important variables to be taken into account in the statistical analyses by incorporating their values as well as subjects' responses to the treatment they receive.

The name ANCOVA indicates that covariates are taken into account in the analysis. A covariate is a variable other than the main variable of interest. In the case of our ongoing example of examining decreases in SBP, subjects' baseline SBP is likely to be of considerable interest. This technique of ANCOVA can be used to control statistically for baseline differences and to prevent them from skewing the results for the treatment effect.

It is quite possible that a subject's baseline SBP and SBP response to the treatment administered may be related. That is, they may covary. For example, one possible scenario is that subjects with very high baseline SBP are more likely to show larger decreases in SBP following treatment than subjects with low baseline SBP values. If this is true, and despite the best intentions of randomization, subjects in one of the treatment groups have notably higher baseline SBP values than those in the other treatment group, and the mean treatment group SBP responses could be impacted by these baseline differences. Analysis of covariance facilitates the following:

- It takes into account chance imbalances that have occurred in a variable despite randomization.
- It gives a more precise estimate of the treatment effect. Some of the variation in the outcome can be ascribed to concomitant variation in the covariate. This allows this variation to be removed from the total error variation against which the effect variation is compared. This means that the denominator in the effect variance/error variance ratio is smaller, making the test statistic calculated of larger magnitude.

The technique of ANCOVA allows more than one covariate to be added to the analysis model. This means that a wide range of variables measured at baseline can potentially be used. While this possibility can initially appear advantageous, it raises a potential concern. Using all of the possible variables is neither practical nor desirable, and so a decision has to be made concerning which ones to include in the ANCOVA model. Importantly, if the covariate is not related to the primary variable of interest, including it in the ANCOVA model is of no benefit.

The best approach is to choose a limited number of covariates that are all related to the outcome variable. The question then becomes: How does one decide on this limited group of related covariates? One strategy would be to look at all baseline values at the end of the trial and to include those that seem very different between the groups in the ANCOVA model. However, this strategy is not ideal. The safest approach is to select "prognostic covariates" before the trial and identify them in the statistical analysis plan (Matthews, 2006). If it is apparent at the end of the planned analysis that another baseline variable is considerably different between groups, this can be included in an identified secondary analysis to explore its effect.

11.4.3 Subgroup Analysis

Subgroup analysis receives a lot of attention in clinical trials. There are various possible explanations for this, some of which are more cynical than others. The response of well-defined subgroups of patients to a therapeutic drug is a topic of legitimate medical interest. It may well be biologically plausible that certain well-defined subgroups would respond differently than other well-defined subgroups, meaning that efficacy and/or safety concerns may be quite different. (Based on our knowledge of the interindividual variation in response to a drug, members of a well-defined subgroup will not all respond identically: The present comments are couched in terms of the typical response of members of a subgroup.) Therefore, it is clinically important to address this question.

From a more cynical viewpoint and a much less statistically justifiable standpoint, there can be temptation to look for any subgroup differences that may exist in a data set and related temptation to be overly enthusiastic about any difference that may surface. This is of particular concern when the overall analysis did not reveal a statistically significant difference between the treatment groups. Matthews (2006) addressed this issue, noting that an important point in subgroup analysis is the question of how the subgroups arose in the first place. Given that the subjects in virtually any clinical trial will exhibit many features that could be used to define subgroups, why and how were the ones of interest selected? Again, if many subgroups are formed and compared, the question of multiplicity will need to be addressed.

Having noted these cautions, subgroup analysis can certainly be meaningful and important. This is particularly so if there is a good biological reason *a priori* to expect that the treatment effects will not be the same in identified subgroups. Also, some unexpected subgroup findings may actually reveal important findings that should be further investigated in additional studies. These observations led Matthews (2006) to distinguish between two sorts of subgroup formation, and hence analysis:

- A limited number of sub-groups identified *a priori* with an apparent biological/clinical reason for the difference of interest.
- Subgroups whose apparent importance is *post hoc* and arises only as a result of doing analyses.

If the treatment effect appears to differ across subgroups identified in the first way, the phenomenon "should be taken much more seriously" that if the subgroups came to light via the second process (Matthews, 2006).

11.4.4 Meta-Analysis

The number of clinical communications published per year has increased to staggering proportions. Matthews (2006) noted that there are currently on the order of 20,000 biomedical journals that publish on the order of two million articles a year. This makes it extremely difficult for a clinician who would like to research a particular topic to locate all of the relevant articles. Accordingly, two kinds of review papers can be very helpful. The first is narrative reviews. These "collate, compare, discuss, and summarize" the current state of knowledge (Matthews, 2006). Narrative reviews are descriptive in nature. The second kind of review incorporates meta-analysis. These reviews are quantitative in nature.

Meta-analysis involves conducting new analyses using previously published results. Published data are combined, therefore creating a larger overall data set and sample size than was the case for any single study. The logic here is that this larger sample size increases the statistical power to detect treatment effects and also allows the magnitude of a treatment effect to be assessed more precisely.

For many reasons, there are likely to be more than one publication that address the same research question. Even when the results are not identical (which is very likely to be the case), consistency in the interpretation of the results is reassuring: Recall the discussion of consistency between ITT and per-protocol analyses in Section 11.2.3. Additionally, results from many smaller studies that are inconclusive can sometimes be combined to paint a picture that is very compelling, and the overall result can be put in a broader context, since it has been attained from different treatment regimens and different subject populations (Matthews, 2006).

Meta-analysis is facilitated by the continuous and enormous increase in computer processing power, data storage capability, and connectivity. As Gad (2006) noted, this electronic availability and accessibility of data "makes it possible to conduct analyses that would be unethical, expensive, or inordinately lengthy to carry out *de novo*." This possibility has an interesting implication for potential new studies. If it is possible to conduct a meta-analysis that will meaningfully answer a research question, there is no good reason to conduct a new trial to answer the question. Accordingly, the Rationale or Justification sections of protocols are increasingly addressing the trial's purpose and addressing the need for the trial on the basis that the research question of interest cannot be answered by a suitable meta-analysis using existing data (Matthews, 2006).

11.5 EQUIVALENCE TRIALS

The goal of equivalence trials is to demonstrate that the test drug and an active comparator drug are equivalent. Like several words that we have already encountered in this book (e.g., significance), the word "equivalent" is used in both everyday language and in Statistics, but its use in Statistics is specific. In this context, equivalence means that, in the "best case scenario," the test treatment is trivially better than the reference treatment and in the "worst case scenario" it is tolerably worse.

When there is already an approved treatment for a disease or condition, a question arises: Why would a new drug that is of "equivalent efficacy" be of interest to clinicians who may prescribe it for their patients? For this to be the case, there need to be other benefits to patients. For example, such reasons may be a lower incidence of side effects or greater dosing convenience, e.g., taking a tablet once a week instead of once a day. Both of these considerations may lead to a better quality of life for a patient. There may be additional benefits to the health care system in general, such as the lower cost of the test drug. This may have implications for personal financing of purchasing the drug and implications for health insurance and reimbursement.

Equivalence trials are also appropriate when the disease being treated is particularly serious (e.g., cancer) and the use of placebo controls would be unethical.

11.5.1 Why the Hypothesis Testing Strategy Is Different Here

The research question in equivalence trials is structured differently from the research question in superiority trials. The hypothesis testing approach that works so well in superiority trials is of little value in an equivalence trial. As Matthews (2006) commented, "Failing to establish that one treatment is superior to the other is not the same as establishing their equivalence."

Imagine that we want to demonstrate that a new drug is as effective as a drug already in widespread use. This comparator drug may have been the first-to-market or it may be acknowledged as the market leader or standard treatment. Such a trial might be designed to demonstrate equivalent efficacy to the standard treatment. In this case, the question of interest is: Does the new drug demonstrate equivalent efficacy compared with the comparator drug? The term "reference drug" is used here to describe the active comparator. This leads to the following research question: Does the new drug demonstrate equivalent efficacy compared with the reference drug?

Given that the format of the research question is different from that used in superiority trials, the formats of the research hypothesis and the null hypothesis are also different. As noted in Section 7.3, the research hypothesis and null hypothesis in superiority trials are stated as follows:

- Research hypothesis: The new drug alters SBP statistically significantly more than the placebo (the reference drug).
- Null hypothesis: The new drug does not alter SBP statistically significantly more than the placebo (the reference drug).

As also noted in Chapter 7, "acceptance" of the research hypothesis is predicated on rejecting the null hypothesis: Recall that the only two options at the end of the hypothesis testing are to reject the null hypothesis or to fail to reject the null hypothesis.

If the hypothesis testing used in superiority trials were employed in equivalence trials, less-than-optimum methodology could result in the "desired result." The null hypothesis used in superiority trials says that there is not a statistically significant difference between the two drugs being compared. In the case of equivalence trials, this is precisely what we are trying to demonstrate. One (accidental) way to dramatically increase the chances of getting a nonsignificant finding in superiority trials is to employ less-than-optimal experimental methodology. Imagine that a superiority trial has been done in a less than optimal way. Imagine that the methodology was poor, e.g., SBP measurements were not made appropriately. What consequences would this have? The lack of appropriate measurement techniques and the consequent poor quality of the SBP data may introduce a lot more error variance than would have been the case had measurement been conducted properly. This additional error variance, even in the presence of a sizeable effect variance (a sizeable treatment size), could lead to a nonsignificant result, which in turn would mean that we would fail to reject the null hypothesis, thereby supporting the statement that the drug and placebo do not differ statistically significantly.

In this scenario, poor methodology could lead to the conclusion that the drug and the placebo do not differ significantly in efficacy. This could have happened even though there was a "real" difference between the drug and the placebo. Underpowering the study could also mean that a sizable treatment effect would not reach statistical significance. This would again lead to failure to reject the null hypothesis, thereby supporting the statement that the drug and placebo do not differ significantly. Therefore, in both cases of less than optimum methodology and less than optimum study design, is it possible that a real difference was not detected. Any occurrence of less-than-optimal design and methodology is not desirable. Under-powering, a design issue, is more understandable than poor methodology. The sample size chosen for the study is provided by sample-size estimation which, by definition, involves the study team making its best estimate in light of the best available evidence (see Chapter 9). In contrast, poor measurement, a methodology issue, is unforgivable. In the case of equivalence trials, we are trying to establish that there is not a statistically significant difference between the new drug and the reference drug. Therefore, we cannot in good faith employ a strategy where less-than-optimum methodology increases the chances of success.

This sentiment is stated more succinctly in ICH E9:

> Concluding equivalence...based on observing a non-significant test result of the null hypothesis that there is no difference between the investigational product and the active comparator is inappropriate (p. 16).

Obtaining a nonsignificant p-value in a superiority trial does not demonstrate that the two treatments are the same. This is an extremely important concept and one that is widely misunderstood. Again, then, obtaining a nonsignificant p-value in a superiority trial does not demonstrate that the two treatments are the same. Conventional p-values have no role in establishing equivalence.

11.5.2 Establishing the Equivalence Margin

Having seen why the hypothesis testing used in superiority trials is inappropriate for equivalence trials, the appropriate approach in this context is now discussed. The first step in this approach is to establish the equivalence margin for the trial.

Consider an equivalence trial to be conducted with the aim of demonstrating that a new drug, represented by "N," is equivalent to an active control agent or reference drug, represented by "R." The primary goal of the trial is to demonstrate that the responses to N and R differ by an amount that is clinically unimportant. The immediate question following this statement is: What is the definition of clinically unimportant? This is decided by the study team on a study-by-study basis. Put another way, the study team has to choose the amount that they will define as clinically unimportant in the context of that trial. This choice may or may not be "right," whatever right is, but it must be made for an equivalence trial to be conducted, and it must be made before the trial data are collected. That is, it must be part of the study design and be documented in the study protocol and/or the statistical analysis plan.

Using the ongoing example of developing a new antihypertensive drug, a study team may decide that a difference of 4 mmHg is "clinically unimportant." (Please note that this is a purely hypothetical value, not based on any actual evidence, and chosen purely for illustrative purposes.) The rationale in this equivalence trial is as follows. If the new drug N has a much better side-effect profile and, in the clinical trial about to be conducted, lowers mean SBP to within 4 mmHg of the mean SBP level achieved by the established drug, R, the new drug N will be declared to have equivalent efficacy. It is then likely that this drug would be chosen over the existing (reference) drug R in clinical practice because it has been declared to have equivalent efficacy and, importantly, it has a better safety profile.

The choice of 4 mmHg permits the construction of the equivalence margins. These margins are defined as ±4 mmHg for this equivalence trial. The trial is then conducted, with all of the necessary attention paid to methodological considerations. At the end of the trial, the data collected are used to calculate the mean SBP change for the new drug treatment group, represented here as ΔN, and the mean SBP change for the reference drug treatment group, represented here as ΔR. (This is done in exactly the same way that would be used if the trial had been a superiority trial testing a drug treatment group and a placebo treatment group.) The treatment effect is then calculated, as in superiority trials, as the difference between the treatment group means.

11.5.3 Hypothesis Construction and Testing

The next step in the case of equivalence trials is quite different from the strategy used in superiority trials. Once the treatment effect has been determined, attention moves directly to calculation of the 95% CI for the treatment effect. Establishing equivalence is based entirely on the use of these CIs. ICH E9 states the following:

> For equivalence trials, two-sided confidence intervals should be used. Equivalence is inferred when the entire confidence interval falls within the equivalence margins (p. 15).

Confidence intervals were introduced in Chapter 8. The CIs discussed there were two-sided, even though this term was not introduced at that time. The term "two-sided" simply means that both the lower and the upper limit of the CI are of interest.

In this case, the research hypothesis states that the two drugs are equivalent, and the null hypothesis states that they are not equivalent. The locations of the lower and the upper limit of the 95% CI determine whether or not the null hypothesis is rejected. If both the lower limit and the upper limit lie within the equivalence margin, we reject the null hypothesis and the new drug and the reference drug are declared to be equivalent. If either the lower limit or the upper limit lies outside the equivalence margin or if both limits lie outside, we fail to reject the null hypotheses, and the drugs are not declared to be equivalent.

11.5.4 Statistical Analysis and Clinical Judgment Working Together

When conducting an equivalence trial, it is necessary to use statistical analysis in conjunction with clinical judgment. The choice of the equivalence margins, which must be made before the trial is conducted, is a clinical judgment. Once the data have been collected, a statistical technique is used to determine if the drugs are to be deemed equivalent. This is a good example of how both statistical thought and clinical thought are necessary in the world of clinical trials.

11.6 NONINFERIORITY TRIALS

Noninferiority trials are very similar to equivalence trials in the manner of their statistical approach. In equivalence trials, a new drug (N) may be of interest, even though an improvement in efficacy is not anticipated, since is has fewer side effects than an existing (reference) drug (R). In the case of noninferiority, we are prepared to go one step further. If the side-effect profile of the new drug *N* is dramatically better than that of the existing drug (R), we may be prepared to accept slightly reduced but noninferior efficacy.

11.6.1 Establishing the Noninferiority Margin

The hypothesis testing approach for noninferiority trials is similar to that used in equivalence trials, as just discussed. The first step in this approach is to establish the noninferiority margin for the trial. Continuing with the theme of using antihypertensive drugs in the examples, imagine a scenario where a new drug N has such a better safety profile compared with the reference drug R that we are prepared to accept a slight decrease in efficacy. The question then becomes: Given this much better safety profile, what decrease in mean efficacy would we accept? This is a clinical question, not a statistical question. The study team must choose this value. This choice may or may not be right, whatever right is, but it must be made in order for a noninferiority trial to be conducted. This decision must be part of the study design.

For the sake of this example, let us say that a decrease in mean efficacy of 3 mmHg in SBP is acceptable. (Please note again that this is a hypothetical example.) The resulting value of minus 3 mmHg yields the noninferiority margin. The trial is then conducted. The treatment effect is calculated, as in superiority trials and equivalence trials, as the difference between the treatment group means.

11.6.2 Hypothesis Construction and Testing

Once the treatment effect has been determined, attention moves directly to calculation of the 95% CI for the treatment effect. As for equivalence trials, *p*-values are not used in noninferiority trials. Establishing noninferiority is based entirely on the use of CIs. ICH E9 states the following:

> For non-inferiority, a one-sided confidence interval should be used.

The term "one-sided confidence interval" arises since attention only needs to be paid to one limit, the lower end, of the 95% CI to investigate noninferiority. Therefore, the other end need not be calculated, and can be left unspecified.

In this case, the research hypothesis states that the test drug is noninferior, and the null hypothesis states that the test drug is not noninferior. The location of the lower limit of the 95% CI determines whether or not the null hypothesis is rejected. If the lower limit falls to the right of the noninferiority margin, we reject the null hypothesis and the new drug N is declared to be non-inferior. If the lower limit falls to the left of the non-inferiority margin, we fail to reject the null hypothesis, and the new drug is not declared to be noninferior.

11.6.3 Statistical Analysis and Clinical Judgment Working Together

As in the case of equivalence trials, it is necessary to use statistical analysis in conjunction with clinical judgment when conducting a noninferiority trial. The choice of the noninferiority margin, which must be made before the trial is conducted, is a clinical judgment. Once the data have been collected, a statistical technique is used to determine whether the new drug is deemed to be noninferior compared with the reference drug.

11.7 BIOEQUIVALENCE STUDIES

Bioequivalence studies are conducted to demonstrate that a new drug has "equivalent" characteristics to an existing drug or that a new formulation of an existing drug has equivalent characteristics to the existing formulation of the drug. Bioequivalence studies can also be used if a new way of administering the drug is thought to be preferable or to be a good alternative in certain situations. The characteristics of interest include both efficacy and safety. If a drug's formulation is altered, data concerning the stability and comparative dissolution of the new formulation are also needed to demonstrate that these changes do not substantially alter the original quality characteristics of the product. Throughout clinical trials, and after marketing approval, changes are often made to the formulation, making bioequivalence testing necessary. There are several places in the drug development process where this can occur:

- Early on when refining the formulation in the pharmaceutics stage.
- Later in the clinical development program to demonstrate that the final commercial formulation to be marketed upon approval is equivalent to the formulation used in confirmatory trials. Issues of mass production and manufacturing scale-up can be relevant here (see Chapter 12).
- When there is a desire for substantial postmarketing formulation alterations.

11.7.1 Use of Cross-Over Designs

Cross-over study designs are typically employed in bioequivalence trials. Imagine that the new formulation is called N and the existing formulation is called R (the reference formulation). The two order possibilities for receiving the two drug treatments are NR and RN. Typically, healthy male and female adults participate in these studies, and the treatment orders are appropriately controlled and balanced. Pharmacokinetic parameters are used to represent both safety and efficacy.

To demonstrate equivalence in plasma concentration profiles, rate and extent of availability must be assessed and compared. The parameters C_{max} and AUC are typically used here, and they are regarded as surrogate markers for clinical safety and efficacy. If they are "too much higher" in the new drug formulation N, they could lead to unwanted side effects. On the other hand, if they are "too much lower," the new formulation may be less effective in treating the condition. The definition of "too much" in this context is not simple, and we will not discuss the details here (see Patterson and Jones, 2006, for more details).

In bioequivalence trials, two hypotheses are set up as follows:

- C_{max} and AUC data for the new formulation N are both too high relative to the reference formulation R.
- C_{max} and AUC data for the new formulation N are both too low relative to the reference formulation R.

In this case, a "double-barreled approach" is taken. Both of these hypotheses need to be rejected in order for N to be deemed bioequivalent to R. If the data lead to the failure to reject one or both of the hypotheses, N is not deemed to be bioequivalent to R (see Hauschke et al., 2007, for additional discussion).

11.8 GROUP SEQUENTIAL DESIGNS

Clinical trials, with almost no exception, are longitudinal (Chow and Liu, 2004). This means that data are accumulated sequentially over time. From the perspective outlined so far in the book, the statistical analysis takes place once the number of subjects stated in the study protocol have been enrolled, randomized, and completed their participation in the trial. This approach can be called the Fixed design or fixed sample design approach. Another design of interest in clinical trials is the group sequential design, in which interim analysis plays a crucial role.

Several interim analyses may be performed during an ongoing clinical trial at various preidentified points. Each interim analysis conducted utilizes all of the data that have been collected to date. The rationale for this approach is that this strategy may reveal compelling evidence that the clinical trial should be stopped at the time of a particular interim analysis because there is already compelling evidence that the drug is effective or that it is toxic. This particular interim analysis could be conducted some considerable time before the trial would have otherwise been completed.

It is important to note here that the word "group" in the name group sequential design does not refer to a treatment group. It refers to the fact that a group of subjects (comprising of subjects from both treatment groups) completes their participation in the study before the initial interim analysis is conducted, a second group of the same number of subjects completes their participation before the second interim analysis is performed, and so on. It is assumed in this methodology that equal (or fairly close to equal) enrollment has occurred in each treatment group at each point that an interim analysis is conducted.

In our ongoing example of developing a new antihypertensive drug, the intervention may be several months long, since it may take this length of time to see the full effect of the drug under investigation. Moreover, such clinical trials typically take much longer to complete than would be suggested simply by considering the length of the treatment period. In a large clinical trial it is not possible to enroll and randomize all of the required subjects on the same day (Chow and Liu, 2004). The duration of a trial is sometimes represented as the time between "first subject first visit" and "last subject last visit," but this does not include planning time, recruitment, screening, and randomization time or the time it takes to analyze the enormous amount of data once they are all collected. It is therefore not unusual for a reasonably large trial to last for several years.

11.8.1 Interim Analyses in Group Sequential Trials

The purpose of interim analyses in group sequential trials is to determine if the clinical trial should be terminated at that point. The rationale for interim analyses of data that are accumulating over time in a clinical trial was established almost 40 years ago, and considerable attention has subsequently focused on the development of statistical approaches and decision-making processes that facilitate the implementation of data monitoring and interim analyses for the early termination of a clinical trial (Chow and Liu, 2004).

One reason for the early termination of a clinical trial would be that the interim analysis provided compelling evidence that the drug under investigation was effective. From an ethical standpoint, this would mean that, if the trial were continued, the subjects in the placebo treatment group would be receiving a placebo for no justifiable reason. One of the central tenets of subject participation in clinical trials is clinical equipoise (see Section 1.8.1), which says that the efficacy of the drug under investigation is not known to be different from placebo, and therefore it is acceptable that some subjects receive a placebo. Once it is known that the drug is effective, it is no longer ethical for some individuals to receive an inferior treatment, and this is the first and foremost reason for terminating the study.

There are also other benefits. From an economic standpoint, a sponsor would save the cost of continuing with the clinical trial, and from a public health standpoint the drug could be approved for marketing earlier, thereby being available to clinicians and patients at an earlier time. A second reason for stopping the trial would be that there is compelling evidence that the trial will not be able to achieve its intended purpose even if it carries on to its maximum number of subjects as specified in the study protocol. A third reason would be that the interim analysis provided compelling evidence that the drug under investigation was harmful.

11.8.2 Data Monitoring Committees

To facilitate interim analyses, a data monitoring process is necessary. This is typically performed by a data monitoring committee (DMC), sometimes called alternative names such as a data and safety monitoring board. Interim monitoring of accumulating data is an area of clinical trials that can be critical to the ethics, efficiency, integrity, and credibility of the trials and their conclusions, and increasingly such monitoring is conducted by formally established committees. The purpose of these committees is "to protect the safety of subjects, the credibility of the study, and the validity of the results" (Ellenberg et al., 2003).

The composition of DMCs is typically multidisciplinary, and the participation of both clinicians and statisticians is critical. The DMC for a particular trial can be appointed by the trial sponsor or by a steering committee. Its duties can include reviewing the initial protocol, monitoring the conduct of the study by assessing accrual, eligibility, protocol compliance, losses to follow-up, and other issues concerned with safeguarding the subjects and the integrity of the trial.

Before a trial starts, a charter needs to be written and agreed upon by the trial sponsor and the committee. This charter describes the structure and operation of the committee and specifies its activities and responsibilities. The DMC should have access to fully unblinded data, with actual treatments and not just codes available for its review. Except in certain limited circumstances, trial integrity is best protected when interim data comparing treatment groups are seen only by the DMC members and statisticians preparing the interim report (Ellenberg et al., 2003, see also O'Neill, 2006).

11.8.3 Statistical Methodology for Interim Analysis

Statistical methods have been developed for interim analysis. Data-dependent stopping rules are established for each trial, stating under what circumstances the results of interim analyses will lead to the early termination of the trial. Data-dependent stopping is the process of evaluating accumulating data in a clinical trial and making a decision whether the trial should be continued or stopped because the available evidence is already convincing (Piantadosi, 2005). These data-dependent stopping rules, along with the number and the timing of planned interim analyses should be stated in the study protocol, just like any other aspect of the study design and methodology, and the statistical procedures to analyze the data at each time point should be specified in the associated statistical analysis plan. Each time an interim analysis is conducted, there will be more data available, since all data collected up to that time point are included in the analysis.

In the fixed sample clinical trial approach, one analysis is performed once all of the data have been collected. The chosen nominal significance level (the Type I error rate) will have been stated in the study protocol and/or the statistical analysis plan. This value is likely to be 0.05: As we have seen, declaring a finding statistically significant is typically done at the 5% *p*-level. In a group sequential clinical trial, the plan is to conduct at least one interim analysis and possibly several of them. This procedure will also be discussed in the trial's study protocol and/or the statistical analysis plan. For example, suppose the plan is to perform a maximum of five analyses (the fifth would have been the only analysis conducted had the trial adopted a fixed sample approach), and it is planned to enroll 1,000 subjects in the trial. The first interim analysis would be conducted after data had been collected for the first fifth of the total sample size, i.e., after 200 subjects. If this analysis provided compelling evidence to terminate the trial, it would be terminated at that point. If compelling evidence to terminate the trial was not obtained, the trial would proceed to the point where two-fifths of the total sample size had been recruited, at which point the second interim analysis would be conducted. All of the accumulated data collected to this point, i.e., the data from all 400 subjects, would be used in this analysis.

Again, if this analysis provided compelling evidence to terminate the trial, it would be terminated at this point. If compelling evidence to terminate the trial was not obtained, the trial would proceed to the point where three-fifths of the total sample size had been recruited, at which point the third interim analysis would be conducted. If this analysis did not provide compelling evidence to terminate the trial, recruitment would continue to 800 subjects, when the fourth interim analysis would take place. If this did not did not provide compelling evidence to terminate the trial, recruitment would continue to the full sample size of 1,000 subjects, when the fifth and final analysis would take place. Regardless of the outcome of this analysis, the trial would terminate at this point, since it was stated in the study protocol that 1,000 subjects was the maximum number that would be recruited.

By its nature, therefore, the group sequential design involves the possibility of multiple testing. In this example it is possible that five analyses could be conducted on data collected in this clinical trial. As discussed in Section 7.10, there is an inherent problem with multiple testing. As more tests are performed, it becomes increasingly likely that a Type I error will occur, i.e., that a result will erroneously be declared as statistically significant. As also noted at that point, however, the problem can be addressed completely satisfactorily by taking appropriate statistical care.

In the context of such interim analysis—repeated analysis to see if the drug response, on average, differs from the placebo response—the same hypothesis is tested five times if the trial is not terminated early and proceeds to its final stage. While the chance of erroneously obtaining a significant result at the 5% level of significance is 1 in 20 if only one analysis is conducted, this chance increases every time more than one test is performed.

One method of addressing the issue of multiple comparisons, the Tukey test conducted after a significant omnibus ANOVA test, was discussed in Section 7.9.3. Another approach to multiple comparisons is the Bonferroni test. The strategy in this case is to divide α (usually 0.05) by the number of tests conducted following a significant omnibus ANOVA test. That is, if three comparisons were to be made, the α-level used for each comparison would become 0.05/3, i.e., 0.017, a more conservative value. While similar in spirit, the approach adopted in group sequential designs differs in its application. First, in the case of these multiple comparisons, it was precisely known before any test was conducted how many multiple comparisons would be made: This was equal to the number of pairs of treatment groups that could be formed. In the case of the Bonferroni test, this provided the number by which the initial α was divided to obtain the appropriately more conservative α-level. In the example of the interim analyses used here, it is not actually known *a priori* how many analyses will be done. The minimum number is one, and the maximum number (which is known *a priori*) is five.

Second, Tukey and Bonferroni multiple comparisons are done at the same point in time, i.e., immediately following a significant omnibus ANOVA result, and, more relevantly, are done with essentially the same amount of data in each case. The actual numbers of subjects in each dose treatment group may be slightly different, but the amounts of data used in each comparison will be very comparable. In contrast, the number of data used in each interim analysis increases linearly from the number used in the previous interim analysis. In our example, the number of data increases from 200 to 400, then to 600, then to 800, and finally to 1,000 if the study is not terminated along the way.

Intuitively, it might be the case that you would put more faith in the results of an analysis conducted on 1,000 subjects, somewhat less in the results of an analysis conducted on 800 subjects, and decreasingly less faith in the results of the other three analyses, respectively. Therefore, there are two statistical considerations to be addressed in the case of interim analyses. First, the fact that more than one analysis may be done increases the probability of a Type I error, and it is therefore appropriate to adjust the α-level in a more conservative direction. Second, it is usual to place more faith in an analysis conducted on a larger sample than on a smaller sample. While there are many statistical approaches to the issue of interim analysis, one notable strategy was suggested by O'Brien and Fleming (see Ellenberg et al., 2003).

The O'Brien-Fleming approach.

This approach modifies the α-level appropriate for each of the individual interim analyses in a trial by considering not only the total number of analyses that may be conducted but also the relative placement of each individual analysis in the string of possible analyses. The O'Brien-Fleming approach effectively makes it considerably harder for the first interim analysis to attain statistical significance, as would a very conservative α-level, and relatively easier for the later ones to attain statistical significance, as would an α-level that approaches the one that would be chosen if there were only one analysis being performed. As Chow and Liu (2004) commented, this means that, when the early interim analyses are conducted on the relatively small amount of data that has been accumulated to date, the results must be extreme to justify recommending termination of the trial. In contrast, when later interim analyses are conducted using a sample size approaching the maximum planned sample size, the statistical criterion for deciding to terminate the study becomes progressively less stringent, approaching the one that would have been chosen for a fixed sample study employing the maximum number of possible participants.

O'Brien and Fleming proposed what has become one of the most widely used group sequential boundaries. In this case, the boundary values are very extreme early in the trial, when the results are still quite unstable. The boundary values become less extreme as the trial progresses, with the critical value at the scheduled final analysis being close to the conventional critical value. This boundary has the desirable property of being very conservative early on when one would be wary of unstable efficacy and safety results.

Group sequential alpha spending functions.

The original methodology for group sequential boundaries required that the number and timing of interim analyses be specified in advance. However, in cases where potentially unfavorable safety data may be emerging, a more flexible implementation of the group sequential boundaries via an alpha spending function may be helpful (see Ellenberg et al., 2003). Waiting the planned 6–12 months for the next look at safety data may not be a good idea if the previous look started to suggest unfavorable data.

An alpha spending function controls how much of the false-positive error, α, is used at each interim analysis such that no more than a predefined maximum can be used altogether. When using an alpha spending function, the only thing that needs to be specified in the study protocol is the particular spending function that has been chosen. The precise number of interim analyses that may be conducted does not need to be specified in advance, and neither does the exact timing of any given analysis. This means that a DMC can start out with a chosen alpha spending function and projected schedule for interim analyses but can then legitimately change the frequency and timing of the analysis as trends emerge as long as the predefined maximum α is not exceeded.

11.8.4 Ethical Considerations in Early Termination

It was noted in Section 5.4 that it is unethical to ask a subject to participate in a clinical trial whose design precludes any useful information being gained from its conduct. This ethical issue has to be addressed before every trial. In the case of trials that may be terminated following interim analysis, ethical considerations need to be addressed for a second time when deciding whether or not to terminate a trial early. Deciding whether or not to terminate the trial on any of the grounds discussed in Section 11.8.1 is not as straightforward as might initially be hoped.

If compelling evidence of efficacy is found in an early interim analysis and the trial is therefore terminated, less safety data will be collected than would have been the case had the trial progressed to its completion. Of particular importance is that data on more prolonged use of the drug are not obtained. This occurrence is less problematic in cases where the drug is a treatment for a life-threatening disease or condition. Here, stopping the trial so that the subjects in the control arm can also be administered the drug may be much more important than prolonging the trial and thus collecting more safety data in the trial itself. Safety data can be collected from the patients as therapy proceeds (the participants in the trial have now become patients under the care of a clinician since they are no longer experimental subjects in a clinical trial).

If it appears that the trial has little chance of demonstrating that the treatment is beneficial, several considerations are pertinent, including:

- Is it likely that this unfavorable trend might reverse itself? If the trial is stopped and the trend would have reversed itself, evidence of treatment benefit that would have been obtained will not be obtained, and that treatment will not reach patients who might have benefited from it.
- While there is little likelihood of statistically demonstrating that the initially anticipated treatment effect will be seen, might it be the case that a smaller treatment effect will emerge that is still clinically significant?

From a statistical point of view, compelling evidence of unexpected adverse events is the hardest to address satisfactorily. When unanticipated safety concerns arise, the fact that they are unanticipated means by definition that they would not have been addressed in the study protocol or statistical analysis plan and that no prespecified analytical strategy is in place. Additionally, the vast range of possible adverse events that might be anticipated means that controlling adequately for multiplicity problems is difficult (Ellenberg et al., 2003).

11.9 ADAPTIVE DESIGNS

Previous sections in this chapter have discussed interim analyses as they are used in group sequential designs. In that strategy, the results of an interim analysis permit the choice of one of two options, terminate the trial or continue the trial, based on the stopping criteria that have been previously stated in the study protocol and/or statistical analysis plan. More recently, however, the results of interim analyses are being used as the basis for other actions, such as changing the endpoints of interest, eliminating certain treatment groups, changing the sample size, or modifying the statistical analysis plan (Liu and Pledger, 2006). Hwang and Lan (2006) made the following observation about the adaptive design approach:

> This allows one to improve expected trial outcomes during the experiment, while still being able to carry out GCP and reach good statistical decisions in a timely fashion. Therefore, adaptive design sometimes can offer significant ethical and cost advantages over standard fixed design (p. 275).

The first time that this approach is encountered, it may appear to run contrary to many of the principles outlined in previous chapters of this book and also to the group sequential methodology outlined earlier in the present chapter. The classical randomized, controlled, fixed sample clinical trial is still a powerful and extremely useful design, and the group sequential methodology is also well established. Nonetheless, there is no doubt that this newer approach of adaptive design is attracting increasing attention.

Three comments are appropriate here. First, consideration of the traditional clinical trial design that has been the focus of attention up until this chapter is extremely worthwhile and instructive: It has facilitated the introduction of fundamental design, methodology, and statistical concepts, and it will be an influential player in pharmaceutical drug development for many years to come. Second, the simple observation that the adaptive design may seem "different" does not in itself make it less valid, less valuable, or less important. Third, statistical approaches that are suitable for adaptive designs are, as yet, less well developed than they are for other study designs.

11.9.1 Protocol Amendments

Historically, clinical trials have often used protocol amendments during the course of a trial. These amendments, which must be approved by an institutional review board just like the original protocol, are made for various reasons. Some examples include modification to the inclusion/exclusion criteria, adjustment of study dose or dose regimen, and the extension of treatment duration. Consider modification to the inclusion/exclusion criteria. If enrollment has been slower than desired, the inclusion/exclusion criteria may be "relaxed" somewhat such that subjects who were close to eligibility originally now become eligible. This process can speed enrollment and bring the trial to completion sooner. This may mean that compelling evidence that the drug is safe and effective is obtained earlier, and the drug becomes available to patients earlier. However, as Chow and Chang (2007) noted:

> If the modifications are made frequently during the conduct of the trial, the target population is in fact a moving target population. In practice, there is a risk that major (or significant) modifications made to the trial and/or statistical procedures could lead to a totally different trial, which cannot address the scientific/medical questions that the trial is intended to answer. Thus, it is of interest to measure the impact of each modification made to the trial procedures and/or statistical procedures after the protocol amendment (p. 44).

Assessing this impact is not straightforward for various reasons, including that, in the case of several protocol amendments, the number of subjects recruited after a given amendment might be quite different than those recruited beforehand. Chow and Chang (2007) therefore strongly recommended that, for good clinical and/or statistical practices, protocol amendments be limited to a small number, such as two or three, in clinical trials.

11.9.2 Increasing Awareness of Adaptive Designs

In one sense, then, the idea of "adapting" the nature of a clinical trial is not new: Regulatory submissions have included trials with protocol amendments for many years. What is relatively new, however, is the recognition that this has indeed been the case (Chow and Chang, 2007). The clinical and statistical implications of such amendments are now receiving considerable interest. Moreover, more "formal" and more sophisticated adaptive strategies and designs are being discussed. Chow and Chang (2007) referred to an adaptive clinical trial design, sometimes called a flexible design, as "a design that allows adaptations or modifications to some aspects (e.g., trial and/or statistical procedures) of the trial after its initiation without undermining the validity and integrity of the trial" (see also Chow et al., 2005).

If appropriate statistical and clinical attention is paid to the adaptations made in an adaptive clinical trial design and to the consequences of these adaptations in the analysis conducted, particularly the statistical inferences and interpretations made, adaptive design can have considerable benefits. It can increase the probability of success for identifying the clinical benefit of the investigative drug, and it can also reflect "real medical practice on the actual patient population with the disease under study" (Chow and Chang, 2007). The latter point is of particular relevance in light of discussions on postmarketing surveillance that follow in Chapter 13. As will be discussed in more detail there, it can be the case that a preapproval clinical trial's rigorous inclusion/exclusion criteria lead to a subject population that does not well reflect the actual patient population with the disease under study. Administration of the drug to this actual patient population, therefore, only occurs after marketing approval when the drug is prescribed by clinicians to "real patients." Therefore, knowledge of the drug's safety and therapeutic benefit in this actual target population is not gained until large-scale postmarketing surveillance is performed. If more knowledge applicable to the actual patient population can be gained in preapproval clinical trials, this is a meaningful advantage.

11.9.3 Regulatory Guidance for Adaptive Designs

Chow and Chang (2007) addressed statistical methodology applicable to various adaptive designs, including adaptive group sequential design, adaptive dose-escalation design, biomarker-adaptive design, adaptive randomization design, adaptive treatment-switching design, and adaptive-hypotheses design. As they noted, however, in the context of drug development there are important regulatory and scientific/statistical questions that need to be addressed:

> Adaptive design methods are very attractive to clinical researchers and/or sponsors due to their flexibility, especially when there are priority changes for budget/resources and timeline constraints, scientific/statistical justifications for study validity and integrity, medical considerations for safety, regulatory concerns for review/approval, and/or business strategies for go/no-go decisions. However, there is little or no information available in regulatory requirements as to what level of flexibility in modifications of trial and/or statistical procedures of on-going trials would be acceptable (p. 44).

While there has been some documentation issued by both European and U.S. regulatory agencies, Chow and Chang (2007) called for regulatory agencies to develop a formal guidance/guideline for adaptive design methods. Clinical scientists and sponsors are interested to know, from a regulatory point of view, the answers to several questions:

- What level of adaptations to the trial and/or statistical procedures would be acceptable?
- How might review and approval processes for adaptive clinical trials differ for different levels of adaptation to trial and/or statistical procedures during a trial?
- Will it be felt that adaptations to a trial and/or statistical procedures have made it more difficult (or even impossible) to address the original study objectives?

Clinical scientists and sponsors also have concerns from the scientific/ statistical point of view. These include:

- Do modifications to clinical trial procedures result in a subject sample from a similar but different target patient population?
- Do modifications of a clinical trial's hypotheses distort the trial's study objectives?
- Does flexibility in statistical procedures employed in a clinical trial lead to biased assessment of the clinical benefit of the investigational drug?

Given the advantages of adaptive designs, there is little doubt that these approaches will continue to receive considerable attention and likely grow in number and sophistication in the relatively near future. Many issues need to be addressed in concert by clinicians, statisticians, clinical scientists, and regulatory reviewers. Further refining the necessary statistical methodology for adaptive designs and optimizing their use in new drug development will be among Statistics' major challenges in the next 5–10 years. At present, adaptive designs are thought to be best suited for early clinical drug development, as opposed to confirmatory therapeutic studies (see Hung et al., 2006).

11.10 BAYESIAN APPROACHES TO ANALYZING CLINICAL TRIALS

Throughout this book, the approach taken to hypothesis testing and statistical analysis has been a "frequentist approach." The name frequentist reflects its derivation from the definition of probability in terms of frequencies of outcomes. While this approach is likely the majority approach at this time, it should be noted here that it is not the only approach. One alternative method of statistical inference is the "Bayesian approach," named for Thomas Bayes' work in the area of probability.

When a clinical trial has been conducted, the frequentist approach we have discussed in the book leads to certain statistical analyses being conducted. A p-value is calculated which provides information leading to the rejection of the null hypothesis or the failure to reject the null hypothesis. Additionally, the analyses lead to an estimate of the treatment effect and its associated confidence intervals. As Spiegelhalter et al. (2004) noted, a Bayesian analysis "supplements this by focusing on how the trial should change our opinion about the treatment effect."

The Bayesian approach forces the researcher to make certain explicit statements:

- A reasonable opinion concerning the plausibility of different values of the treatment effect *excluding* the evidence obtained from the trial in question. This is known as the "prior" probability distribution.
- The support for different values of the treatment effect based *solely* on data from the trial. This is known as the "likelihood."
- A final opinion about the treatment effect. This opinion is the result of combining the previous two sources, and it is known as the "posterior" probability distribution.

The final combination represented in the third statement is performed using Bayes theorem, which "essentially weights the likelihood from the trial with the relative plausibilities defined by the prior distribution" (Spiegelhalter et al., 2004).

Some investigators have argued strongly that one approach is more "appropriate" than the other, while others have argued equally passionately in the opposite direction. What seems more likely is that both approaches can make valuable contributions in the domain of clinical trials. It is likely that the refinement of existing statistical methodologies and the development of new ones will be a very important aspect in the future evolution of clinical trial methodology.

For a good introduction to Bayesian approaches to clinical trials, see Spiegelhalter et al. (2004). See also Piantadosi (2005) for useful discussion of different philosophies of statistical thought.

12

Pharmaceutical and Biopharmaceutical Drug Manufacturing

12.1 Introduction

As noted in Section 3.2.3, drug discovery/design pays close attention to the pharmacokinetics of a drug candidate. A drug molecule with a good pharmacodynamic profile, i.e., a profile that indicates it would interact successfully with its target receptor, will not be clinically useful if it does not reach the target receptor in the chemical state necessary to affect a response. Therefore, getting the drug to the microenvironment of the target receptor in the necessary chemical state is a key consideration. In addition to pharmacokinetic considerations, pharmaceutical considerations are critical (recall Section 3.2.4). Successfully producing, or manufacturing, the drug candidate for nonclinical testing and clinical trials and manufacturing the drug for postapproval marketing are critical. Moreover, their complexity and difficulty should not be underestimated.

When it is thought that the drug molecule can survive the journey from the site of administration to the vicinity of the target receptor, enough of the drug candidate has to be produced for each stage of testing. The drug candidate has to be administered in a certain manner (e.g., a tablet or an injection), and the method of administration has to be determined and developed. In blinded comparative trials, the comparator drug (placebo or active drug) also has to be identified, and both the drug candidate and the comparator drug produced in a manner that allows blinding.

If all goes well in the therapeutic confirmatory trials and the drug is approved, successful commercialization of the approved drug has its own demands. Of relevance in this chapter is the sponsor's ability to manufacture sufficient quantities of the drug in a form that can be readily transported from the manufacturing plant to the pharmacy and in a form that demonstrates stability and therefore has a suitably long shelf-life.

As noted in Section 1.9, pharmaceutical and biopharmaceutical manufacturing processes differ according to the stage of new drug development. Initially, very small amounts of the drug are needed, and this "manufacturing" typically occurs on a laboratory scale. The amount of drug candidate needed becomes progressively larger as the clinical development program proceeds. Eventually, once the drug is approved by a regulatory agency, full-scale commercial manufacturing is needed. It was also noted in Section 1.9 that the transition from small-scale production to commercial-scale manufacturing is far more complex than simply building proportionately larger manufacturing equipment. For example, many laboratory-scale manufacturing processes in the biopharmaceutical arena cannot be easily

New Drug Development: Design, Methodology, and Analysis. By J. Rick Turner

scaled or proportionally increased to produce commercially useful quantities of the drug, and different instruments and analytical techniques are needed (Ho and Gibaldi, 2003).

While this is a brief chapter, it is appropriate to overview the manufacturing of pharmaceuticals and biopharmaceuticals in the context of this book, since effective medications will not be useful unless they are available to clinicians and their patients.

12.2 NONCLINICAL DEVELOPMENT

In early phases of nonclinical development, relatively smaller amounts of the drug product (test materials) are needed, and the immediate focus of manufacturing attention is on small-scale synthesis of the drug substance. At this stage, the quantities needed are in the gram range. Studies do not need to be conducted to cGLP standards, and the drug compound does not need to be manufactured to cGMP standards. However, both cGLP and cGMP standards must be met by later nonclinical studies. Therefore, the drug compound for these toxicological evaluations has to be identical in terms of quality and characteristics to the substance that is administered to humans (Rang, 2006b).

Given the expense of producing test material that meets cGMP standards, chronic toxicological work is typically not started until the drug has been prepared to this standard for the commencement of clinical trials.

12.3 DRUG PRODUCTS FOR CLINICAL TRIALS

As a drug development program moves toward the commencement of clinical trials, the production of clinical drug products needs to be addressed. These clinical drug products include both the new investigative drug and the control materials, i.e., a placebo or an active comparator drug that will be administered to the control group. These materials need to be manufactured in a way that facilitates the blinding that is a hallmark of blinded, concurrently controlled, randomized clinical trials.

12.3.1 Need for the Investigative Drug and the Control Drug

The sponsor is in full control of manufacturing the investigational new drug, since the sponsor "owns" it. If the control drug is a placebo or an active comparator owned by the sponsor, the sponsor is also in full control of this manufacturing process. However, if the active comparator contains another company's active pharmaceutical ingredient (API), permission from that company will be needed.

The use of an active comparator (regardless of its manufacturer) also raises another issue. It is conventional that the active comparator chosen is the "gold standard" of care at the time. However, this simple statement belies the complexity of defining the gold standard in each case. Brun (2006) raised the following questions in this regard:

- Is the gold standard the medication with the highest sales figures?
- Is it the medication with the best reputation among physicians? (This criterion raises the question of how "reputation" is best quantified.)
- Are there different gold standards in different countries? If so, which one should be chosen in multicenter trials being conducted in countries with differing views?

While the choice of the comparator drug to be employed is a joint decision involving clinical and medical groups, regulatory affairs, the clinical supplies group, and the purchasing department, the final decision may well be governed by the accessibility of prime candidates. If the sponsor does not own the comparator drug, comparator medication can sometimes conveniently be purchased from the parent company under a reciprocal arrangement, but it can also be a more complicated process. The comparator drug's company may wish to inspect the study protocol before making a decision, which could involve the test drug's company divulging proprietary information. The comparator drug's company may be concerned about the amount of drug requested, especially if it foresees any shortage due to likely increased demand during the time of its commitment to provide its drug. An additional complexity here is that a detailed agreement and arrangement needs to be made concerning the action to be taken if the comparator drug is recalled (Brun, 2006).

12.3.2 Blinding of Drug Products for Clinical Trials

In addition to manufacturing both the test drug and the comparator drug, these materials need to be blinded. A trial may be called a double-blind study when neither the subjects nor any of the people concerned with their evaluation and care know which treatment the subjects are receiving. While double-blind trials predominate, in some cases a single-blind trial is conducted if it is not possible to blind the subjects (or sometimes the investigators). When trials are conducted in which everyone knows what treatment a subject is receiving, the trial is said to be unblinded.

Blinding makes the drug product and the comparator product look (smell, taste, etc.) the same. In a sizable drug development program, the clinical drug products needed for some of the trials may be different from those used in other trials, since dosage and formulation may change over time as the drug development program proceeds. Thus, even though the same new drug molecule is being investigated, several clinical drug products may need to be manufactured.

The blinding of clinical drug products for double-blind trials involves two steps: making the test drug and the comparator drug as similar as possible in appearance (e.g., color and shape, if they are tablets) and other pertinent characteristics (e.g., taste and smell) and then packaging them in such a way that they cannot be distinguished by the package in which they are supplied to investigators. This process is contrary to the manner in which marketed drugs are supplied. As specified in cGMP guidelines, all marketed drugs need to be manufactured and packaged such that they are clearly identifiable. Therefore, the manufacture and supply of clinical drug products requires special attention.

While a relatively small amount of clinical drug products may be required for early-phase trials, later-phase trials can require considerable amounts, and therefore their manufacture is not a trivial undertaking. Also, while the majority of blinded trials are conducted using solid dosage forms, blinding can also be needed for other drug forms, such as oral liquid formulations, injectable solutions, ointments, and metered dose inhalers (Brun, 2006). Since protein biopharmaceuticals are typically administered by injection, manufacturing clinical drug products in this case can be a challenge.

The most common method of blinding solid dosage forms is over-encapsulation into opaque, hard gelatine capsules. An inactive filler material is used to fill any excess space once the drug being blinded has been placed inside the capsule. When employing this methodology, comparative dissolution testing is necessary, since the over-encapsulation is a modification of the drug (Brun, 2006).

12.3.3 Packaging and Distributing Clinical Drug Products

As noted, clinical drug products then need to be packaged in a special way that is quite different from that employed for commercially available drugs: The content of a package that contains clinical drug products cannot be deduced from the package itself. This presents special challenges in this arena (see Dolfini and Tiano, 2006). Once packaged, clinical drug products need to be distributed to all of the investigational sites participating in a trial. Given that many multicenter trials may now use sites in various countries, this adds several degrees of potential complexity to the process. If international shipping is required, each country's Customs (import/export) authorities may need to be appraised of the drug products' entry into that country.

12.4 COMMERCIAL MANUFACTURING

Monkhouse (2006a) made the following illuminative comments in the context of the difficulties of preparing for commercial-scale manufacturing:

> The difficulty of converting a laboratory concept into a consistent and well-characterized medical product that can be mass-produced has been highly under-rated. Problems in physical

> design, characterization, manufacturing scale-up, and quality control routinely derail or delay development programs (p.2).

Not surprisingly, pharmaceutical companies want to start selling their new drugs as soon as possible following regulatory approval to do so. The sale of drugs provides the financing for future research and development of other drugs as well as for personnel, office buildings, and all the other necessary costs of running a for-profit business. This can lead to a desire to make the transition from laboratory-scale manufacturing to commercial-scale manufacturing by simply increasing the size of each component of the manufacturing process in a linear fashion. However, this rarely works well. While initially more expensive, it is typically a better long-term, cost-effective strategy to develop manufacturing processes and facilities specifically suited for the required demand.

12.5 QUALITY CONTROL: BUILDING QUALITY INTO THE PROCESS

Conventional batch pharmaceutical manufacturing has often been very inefficient (Monkhouse, 2006b). Historically, manufacturing practice involved completing a certain part of the overall process and then taking samples for quality testing. This meant that production was halted until the results of the quality testing were known, which in turn meant that expensive equipment often sat idle and a lot of (paid) personnel time was not productively used. In a multiphase process, this led to constant sampling and the consequent waiting for laboratory analysis of the samples before being given the go-ahead to continue. If the analysis revealed that the samples had not attained the necessary levels of quality, that batch of intermediate product would have to be reprocessed or possibly discarded. In both scenarios, time and resources were not used efficiently.

A more efficient approach is to design quality into the manufacturing process rather than post-testing the finished product. The use of automation and continuous process monitoring involves measuring product attributes in real time and adjusting process operating parameters via feedback/feedforward controls to make necessary adjustments during the manufacturing steps. This strategy can substantially decrease the need for reworks.

For real-time monitoring and control of manufacturing processes, a high degree of knowledge about the desired characteristics of the product and the individual components of the manufacturing process is needed. This knowledge allows hardware and software engineers and programmers to design, test, and implement the necessary control systems, including complex algorithms that utilize many variables. Multivariate statistical analysis is therefore an integral component of these systems. Statistical approaches are also integral to methods such as Six Sigma (e.g., see El-Haik and Al-Aomar, 2006) that help engineers and quality professionals improve manufacturing processes (Monkhouse, 2006b).

12.6 STABILITY STUDIES

Tsong et al. (2006) defined the stability of a drug product as its capacity "to remain within the established acceptance criteria to ensure its identity, strength, quality, and purity within a specified period of time." Stability testing permits the determination of the length of time that the drug product is expected to remain within the approved acceptance criteria as long as the drug product has been stored as stated on the container label. At the manufacturing facility, an expiration date is placed on the package that contains the drug, stating the date after which the drug should not be used. In this manner, the shelf-life of the drug is communicated. The reason for the shelf-life is that, once manufactured, drug products are exposed to many environmental conditions—notably light, temperature, and humidity—that can lead to their chemical decomposition (Florence and Attwood, 2006). Therefore, it is important to know how well the drug product withstands these potential assaults. This is the domain of stability testing.

Statistics plays an important role in estimation of the shelf-life and therefore in the determination of the expiration date placed on each batch of manufactured drug product. Stability testing is an expensive undertaking, and one that is made more complex when a given drug is produced in various dosages and also possibly packaged in various formats. Regulatory agencies require that stability testing must be performed for a minimum of three batches, a number that is reasonably low but still permits statistical analysis of interbatch variability.

Tsong et al. (2006) outlined one simple strategy for stability testing. A number of containers from a production batch are placed in storage at specified conditions. These are chosen to reflect the typical conditions in which the drug product will be stored in regular patient use. Samples are then taken and tested at certain specified intervals (e.g., every three to six months), at which times the drug product's physical, chemical, and biological attributes are evaluated. The FDA and many pharmaceutical companies currently use a statistical technique called linear regression to analyze long-term stability data, although several more complex approaches are possible (see Tsong et al, 2006). ICH Guidelines Q1E and Q1A(R2) also provide guidance for design, methodology, and analysis in stability studies.

12.7 IMMEDIATE RELEASE AND MODIFIED RELEASE TABLETS AND CAPSULES

Tablets and capsules can be manufactured in different ways that release the active pharmaceutical ingredient at different rates. The main categories are:

- Immediate release.
- Modified release.

Immediate release tablets are formulated to release the (API) as soon as possible to hasten absorption. Modified release formulations release the API at a controlled rate. Modified release formulations can be classified into controlled release and extended release formulations. The intention of these formulations is to allow a reduction in dosing frequency or diminish the fluctuation of drug levels on repeated administration compared with that observed with the immediate release form of the drug.

12.8 PRODUCING RECOMBINANT PROTEIN BIOPHARMACEUTICALS

As for small-molecule drug development, proteins and polypeptide-based new molecular entities that demonstrate desirable pharmacological activities move forward to nonclinical testing in appropriate animal models to characterize *in vivo* pharmacokinetics and toxicology. At this point, it is necessary to produce the drug candidate in quantities of milligrams to grams: This is considerably more than the micrograms produced on a laboratory scale during the discovery phase (Ho and Gibaldi, 2003). Larger scale "manufacture" involves the use of genetically engineered host cells with maximum efficiency in producing proteins that are safe and effective (Ho and Gibaldi, 2003).

One possibility is to use prokaryotic cells. These cells are lower organisms (including bacteria) in which DNA is not organized into chromosomes. For equal rates of production yield of recombinant protein and similar purification costs, prokaryotic cells with the highest growth rate should theoretically be a less expensive way to produce the desired protein than eukaryotic cells (which have chromosomal DNA: recall discussions in Section 3.6). Prokaryotic cells proliferate more rapidly. In some instances, however, eukaryotic cells are necessary as the host cells. Lower eukaryotic cells such as yeast can be used where appropriate, while higher eukaryotic cells (mammalian cells) are used where necessary. In these cases, the cost of production typically exceeds $1 million per kilogram (Ho and Gibaldi, 2003).

The use of prokaryote host cells (a less expensive option), lower eukaryote cells (of intermediate cost), or mammalian cells (as just noted, more than $1 million per kilogram) is predicated on what kind of host cell is needed to best express the recombinant protein. Prokaryotes such as *E. coli* cannot carry out post-translational modifications (see Section 14.8.2) such as glycosylation, which can limit their usefulness in producing certain therapeutically useful proteins: Many such proteins are glycosylated (i.e., they are glycoproteins) when they are produced naturally in the body (Walsh, 2003). Glycoproteins have a range of biological activities, including two of particular relevance in this book's discussions: They act as receptors and enzymes.

As Walsh (2003) noted, yeast cells (particularly *Saccharomyces cerevisiae*) have several characteristics that make them useful production systems for recombinant biopharmaceuticals:

- Their molecular biology has been studied in detail, providing information that facilitates genetic manipulation.
- They have a long history of industrial applications in brewing and baking, and many of them are "'generally regarded as safe" (GRAS).
- They grow relatively quickly in relatively inexpensive media.
- Their tough outer cell wall protects them from physical damage.
- They can carry out post-translational modifications of proteins, but while the products resemble the products of human cells, they are not identical.
- The technology for their use, industrial-scale fermentation equipment, is already available (see Section 12.8.1).

Approved therapeutic proteins are used in various conditions, including diabetes, bone marrow transplantation, and vaccination.

The genetic manipulation of animal cells allows the production of therapeutic proteins in animal cell culture systems. Mammalian cells such as Chinese hamster ovarian cells and baby hamster kidney cells are commonly used. These mammalian hosts produce recombinant proteins that have almost identical properties to those made by human cells. However, the use of mammalian cells does have disadvantages. As noted earlier, they are expensive to use. This is influenced by their more complex nutritional requirements, their slower growth, and their increased susceptibility to physical damage (Walsh, 2003).

12.8.1 Commercial-Scale Manufacturing

The process of fermentation is used in various industrial settings, including the production of protein biopharmaceuticals. This process involves growing cells and microbes for the production of the desired product in large quantities under well-specified conditions. Fermentation procedures are typically optimized in a systematic manner in a pilot plant with a fermentor with a capacity on the order of 30 liters, and engineers determine the best strategies to develop fermentors with a capacity on the order of 100,000 liters (Ho and Gibaldi, 2003).

Fermentation can only be used for cells that can grow in suspension. This includes most prokaryotes (including *E. coli*) and lower eukaryotes (including yeast) but only a small percentage of mammalian cells. Most recombinant mammalian cells require a surface support to replicate. These cells, known as adherence cells, are typically grown in roller bottles.

Production of protein biopharmaceuticals synthesized in recombinant prokaryotic or eukaryotic cells can be divided into three stages (Walsh, 2003):

- Upstream processing: The fermentation process that initially generates the product.
- Downstream processing: Purification of the protein product and placing the product into the finished format. This includes filling the product into its containers and sealing the containers.
- Labeling and packaging.

Downstream processing involves employment of a purifying system that can isolate the product in as few steps as possible using the simplest purification technology that will achieve the required purity. While purity is a critical consideration for both small-molecule pharmaceuticals and biopharmaceuticals, the nature of biopharmaceutical administration (typically via injection) and the nature of biotechnology processes require that additional considerations be paid to the purity of biopharmaceuticals. The final product must meet regulatory purity and sterility standards and must be below the maximally acceptable cellular or microbial contamination (Ho and Gibaldi, 2003).

Readers are referred to Ho and Gibaldi (2003), Ng (2004), and Walsh (2003) for further discussion of biopharmaceutical manufacturing and GMP.

13

Postmarketing Surveillance and Evidence-Based Medicine

13.1 Introduction

The fundamental importance of safety assessment throughout the drug development process has been emphasized many times in previous chapters. These chapters have discussed "engineering safety" into new molecular entities, safety evaluations in nonclinical studies, and safety evaluations in clinical trials. Pharmacokinetic and pharmacodynamic assessments, consideration of side effect profiles, and examination of laboratory data all play a critical role in safety assessment of a new investigational drug. Efficacy is also considered throughout the drug development process, particularly in the discovery phase and then again in therapeutic exploratory and therapeutic confirmatory clinical trials.

However, it must be noted at this stage of the book that these assessments of safety and efficacy have their limitations. As Olsson and Meyboom (2006) noted:

> The randomized controlled clinical trial is the method of choice for the objective and quantitative demonstration of the efficacy and tolerability of a new medicine. None the less, such studies have limitations in discovering possible adverse events that may occur, in particular those that are rare or develop after prolonged use, in combination with other drugs, or perhaps due to unidentified risk factors. Clinical trials are inherently limited in duration and number of patients, and, significantly, patients are selected prior to inclusion. In other words, the conditions of a trial are artificial compared with the real-life use after the introduction of a medicine (p. 229).

This statement may sound somewhat surprising, since randomized clinical trials have been a major focus of the book until now. However, the strength of randomized clinical trials is that they are comparative, not necessarily representative (see Senn, 1997). From this point forward, it may be helpful to think of the clinical trials we have discussed so far as preapproval clinical trials, i.e., clinical trials whose results are reported in regulatory applications for marketing approval. These preapproval trials are essential to the process of new drug development, but it is extremely important to realize that evaluation of a drug must not stop once marketing approval has been granted. The title of this part of the book, Lifecycle Clinical Development, makes the point that the drug must be evaluated throughout its lifecycle.

This chapter therefore focuses on monitoring activities that occur following the drug's approval for marketing by a regulatory agency. The chapter discusses the collection of broad-based evidence concerning a drug's safety and therapeutic benefit when the drug is being taken by a large number of individuals in the target patient population. In this context, the term "effectiveness" is used instead of the term "efficacy": Efficacy refers to assessments of therapeutic benefits in preapproval clinical trials.

It should also be noted that "postapproval" clinical trials can be conducted as experimental means of collecting further information about the drug. While these trials can be very informative, the focus of this chapter is on wide-ranging postmarketing surveillance (see Buncher and Tsay, 2006b).

13.2 LIMITATIONS OF PREAPPROVAL CLINICAL TRIALS

While preapproval clinical trials are crucial in drug development, even the gold standard double-blind, randomized, concurrently controlled clinical trials are limited in their ability to provide information that truly represents the safety and effectiveness of the drug once it has been widely prescribed and is being taken by many more individuals than participated in the preapproval clinical trials.

Several issues are pertinent here. One issue is the (very) low probability of observing rare adverse events in clinical trials, even in large therapeutic confirmatory trials. Rare side effects are probabilistically much more likely to surface once the drug is widely used, and unfortunately some of these side effects may be extremely serious. A second issue concerns the fact that clinical trials typically employ relatively homogeneous subject samples. It was noted in Section 10.12 that the inclusion and exclusion criteria (recall also Section 5.7.1) that are used in clinical trials can be extensive, and they usually mean that the subject population in a trial is relatively homogenous. For example, potential subjects who have other illnesses or medical conditions, including renal and hepatic impairment, are typically excluded. The age range of subjects can be fairly limited, and potential subjects taking certain concomitant medications may be excluded from the trial. A third issue concerns the length of time that a patient may take the new drug: This may be considerably longer than the treatment period for subjects in preapproval clinical trials. The long-term safety of a drug that is suitable for chronic administration is therefore not fully known at the time that the drug is approved. Additionally, its propensity for abuse is not known, nor is the likelihood that patients will develop a dependency on the drug.

Another important point concerns how drugs are actually taken by patients. There are considerable challenges to conceptualizing and measuring regimen adherence (Bosworth et al., 2006a). Accordingly, research reviews find widely ranging rates of adherence. An average figure of 50% adherence is not unreasonable (Bosworth et al., 2006a). Improving adherence rates to drug regimens is of vital importance (see Bond, 2004).

Various issues, therefore, limit the generalizability of preapproval clinical trial results. The actual safety and efficacy of the drug in the specific subjects employed in a given clinical trial are certainly of considerable interest, but of much more interest are the likely safety and effectiveness of the drug once it is taken by many members of the target population. Therefore, additional drug monitoring is necessary. This is the province of postmarketing surveillance. This chapter discusses the collection of evidence concerning a drug's safety and effectiveness in its target patient population.

13.2.1 The "Art" of Defining a Study Population in Preapproval Clinical Trials

It is somewhat of an art, albeit a very important one, to carefully define a study population so that a new treatment can be shown to be effective but not so carefully that the treatment effects are not applicable to more heterogeneous populations. It is a balancing act to optimize design in early studies to demonstrate an effect but to make sure that later studies are not so optimized that their results do not generalize well (see Friedman et al., 2006, for additional discussion of generalization).

13.3 POSTMARKETING SURVEILLANCE

A cohort study is a nonexperimental study (recall Section 5.5 for discussion of experimental and nonexperimental studies) that collects information from an identified group of individuals in an overall population. Cohort studies are used widely in epidemiology and clinical epidemiology, and, as Haynes et al. (2006) noted, "evidence from cohort studies (also known as cohort analytical studies) is the next most powerful method after the controlled trial" (see also Fletcher and Fletcher, 2005; Webb et al, 2005; Woodward, 2005).

A group of individuals of particular interest in this context is comprised of patients who are receiving a specific drug. Campbell and Machin (1999) noted that "postmarketing surveillance is a particular type of cohort study carried out on a population of people receiving an established drug." A widely used new drug may be monitored for any untoward medical event happening to patients receiving the drug. In addition to collecting this information, the incidence of advents events with the new drug may be compared with the incidence in patients receiving alternatives to the new drug.

Postmarketing surveillance requires the reporting of relevant information, collating reports from all sources, conducting formal epidemiological studies, and disseminating this information to health professionals. This process is crucial to public safety and public health. In many ways, the information gathered once the drug has been marketed and is in widespread use is likely the most useful to clinicians, but it takes a while for this information to be collected and collated. One key aspect of postmarketing surveillance focuses on safety data, and remaining vigilant for any evidence of side effects not seen in the preapproval clinical trials. A second concerns the fact that the drug may be considered by clinicians for individuals in special populations that may not have been well represented in those clinical trials. Collecting safety data from any of these patients may prove particularly informative in monitoring the overall safety profile of the drug. In addition to safety monitoring, it is also important to note that postmarketing data concerning the drug's therapeutic usefulness can be instructive in terms of further refining the drug's pharmacotherapeutic profile.

Relatedly, once a drug has been marketed and has proved to be successful (clinically successful as indicated in published clinical communications and likely commercially successful as evidenced by annual sales reports), other companies may wish to develop similar products that they feel will have a clinical (and commercial) advantage. This process involves the development of an analog of the established drug (see Fischer and Ganellin, 2006).

Pharmacovigilance is "a search for the unexpected," and its ultimate goal is "the promotion of rational and safe use of medicines" (Olsson and Meyboom, 2006). This goal is facilitated by various activities, including:

- Detecting any new adverse reactions or other important drug-related problems as soon as possible.
- Quantification of any identified issues.
- Benefit/harm evaluation.
- Dissemination of information and education.

There are innumerable reasons why the administration of a drug can lead to unexpected occurrences, some of which may be harmful. For example, hypersensitivity reactions may occur. These reactions may only show up in 1 in 10,000, meaning that they would be probabilistically unlikely to have been seen in pre-approval clinical trials, and they may show "a remarkable absence of a relationship between dose and severity" (Olsson and Meyboom, 2006). The underlying mechanism for this reaction may be an inborn variation in metabolism, but in many cases the etiology is unknown. Another example is therapeutic ineffectiveness. Therapeutic ineffectiveness is not often considered to be a side-effect, but it is one of the most common unintended responses to a drug. It is a recognized reportable event in pharmacovigilance, especially when it occurs unexpectedly (Olsson and Meyboom, 2006).

Interactions with other drugs or with food or herbal preparations are another potential cause of unexpected occurrences. While this has not been discussed in this book, the ever-present issue of potential interactions between drugs taken concomitantly is a critically important one. The FDA issued a draft guidance in September 2006 entitled "Drug Interaction Studies—Study Design, Data Analysis, and Implications for Dosing and Labeling," which is a rich source of information in this area (see also Hansten, 2004).

Inappropriate use of a drug can be a major cause of unexpected occurrences. Acute medication errors are unfortunately higher than may be initially thought. The potential for chronic inappropriate drug use, particularly as it relates to dependence, is also of concern. All of these issues are of interest in pharmacovigilance. After marketing approval for a new drug has been received, the sponsor must review all safety data it obtains from any source worldwide, including:

- Commercial marketing experience.
- Postmarketing clinical investigations.
- Postmarketing epidemiological/surveillance studies.
- Reports in published scientific literature.
- Reports in unpublished papers (as available).

13.3.1 The 2005 CDER Report to the Nation

The FDA's 2005 CDER Report to the Nation, "Improving Public Health Through Human Drugs," is a far-reaching report that is excellent reading for everyone interested in new drug development, containing informative discussions on many aspects of the CDER's activities. Of relevance to this section of the book are the CDER's drug safety activities, particularly the CDER's role in drug safety oversight and surveillance of the safety of products sold in the United States.

The report noted that, during this time, the CDER processed and evaluated "more than 460,000 reports of adverse drug events, including more than 25,000 submitted directly from individual health-care providers and patients." In addition to this ongoing work, the CDER's new initiatives included:

- Establishing a Drug Safety Oversight Board. In its initial meetings, board members explored the methods used in risk assessment of marketed drugs, including review and analysis of spontaneous reports of adverse events, drug use data, health-care administrative data, epidemiological and nonexperimental studies, postapproval clinical trials, and active surveillance systems.
- Sharing drug safety information sooner and more broadly.
- Laying the foundations of an electronic information infrastructure that will give patients, health-care professionals, and consumers quick and easy access to the most up-to-date and accurate information on medicines.
- Obtaining public input on their drug risk communication strategies.

13.4 THE INSTITUTE OF MEDICINE'S 2006 REPORT ON DRUG SAFETY

The Institute of Medicine (IOM) of the National Academies is a not-for-profit organization that was chartered in 1970 as a component of the National Academy of Sciences. It publishes reports on many topics in the fields of biomedical science, medicine, and health (see http:/www.iom.edu). In September 2006, the IOM's Committee on the Assessment of the U.S. Drug Safety System issued a report, commissioned by FDA, entitled "The Future of Drug Safety: Promoting and Protecting the Health of the Public." The report offered a broad set of recommendations to ensure that consideration of safety extends from before product approval through the entire time the product is marketed and used. These recommendations included:

- Clarification of the FDA's authority and additional enforcement tools for the agency.
- Clarification of the FDA's role in gathering and communicating additional information on marketed products' risks and benefits.
- Mandatory registration of clinical trial results to facilitate public access to drug safety information.
- An increased role for the FDA's drug safety staff.
- A large boost in funding and staffing for the agency.

It is currently somewhat paradoxical that the "best" information about a drug's safety and effectiveness is gathered postmarketing, and yet regulatory governance of the collection and dissemination of this information is considerably less than the regulatory governance of premarketing nonclinical and clinical research. Integrated and equally stringent regulatory governance throughout a drug's lifecycle is a worthwhile goal. The IOM report notes that the FDA's critical mission, to protect and advance the public's health, requires that it be given adequate resources (financial and personnel) and authority to enforce defined penalties and sanctions in the domain of post-marketing evaluation of a drug's safety.

13.5 EFFECTIVENESS

While drug safety is extremely important in postmarketing surveillance, it is also of great interest to investigate a drug's effectiveness. Another paradox in the clinical development arena is that the (desirable) nature of tightly controlled preapproval clinical trials, while necessary and informative in its own way, limits the generalizability of the therapeutic results obtained to interventional therapy outside that setting. Extensive inclusion and exclusion criteria mean that these trials evaluate efficacy in a narrow segment of the ultimate target population. From one statistical perspective, this tightly controlled subject population is beneficial since it reduces extraneous variation that may lead to a treatment effect being difficult to detect. These rigorous trials are necessary to address the biological importance of the drug's pharmacodynamic profile, i.e., its efficacy. However, a clinically important biological effect seen in well-controlled trials may not be reflected in the drug's widespread therapeutic profile. This is why effectiveness assessments are needed. Effectiveness trials, or large-scale trials (Piantadosi, 2005), typically employ simple methods of assessment and data capture. They collect data from a large number of patients from heterogeneous populations.

13.6 PUBLISHING CLINICAL RESEARCH IN PEER-REVIEWED CLINICAL JOURNALS

In addition to preparing and submitting documentation to regulatory agencies, the results of clinical studies are reported to the scientific and clinical communities via clinical communications published in medical journals. It was noted in Chapter 1 that presenting the results of a clinical study to the clinical community falls under the scope of this book's expanded definition of Statistics. This section briefly reviews the skills necessary to write good clinical publications and also introduces the peer-reviewed publishing process.

13.6.1 The Peer-Review Process

Leading journals (in clinical and many other realms of scientific inquiry) use a peer-review process when deciding whether or not to accept a paper submitted for publication. A journal's editor, to whom a submission is sent, will typically assign responsibility for the paper's review to an associate editor. This editor will then send the submission to a small group of scientists who are engaged in the same field of investigation as the authors of the submitted paper. These scientists are the peers of the authors, and hence the term peer reviewed. While certainly not perfect, the peer-review system is regarded as the best system for ensuring that high-quality papers are accepted by journals for publication. Papers published in peer-reviewed journals carry much more weight than publications in sources that are not peer reviewed.

During the peer-review process, reviewers evaluate the submission, provide comments, and make a recommendation concerning its suitability for publication. Their identity is typically not revealed to the authors of the submission when their comments and recommendations are forwarded to the authors (and sometimes the reviewers do not know who wrote the paper they are reviewing). Typical recommendations are:

- Publish "as is" (a very rare occurrence).
- Publish with minor revisions.
- Rereview after revision of the paper according to suggestions made by the reviewer.
- Reject the submission.

The associate editor collates the comments from each of the reviewers and sends these back to the authors, who then respond by submitting a revised manuscript (unless the paper has been rejected). The paper may be accepted upon resubmission, sent back for further revision, or rejected if reviewers' comments have not been addressed to the satisfaction of the associate editor.

13.6.2 Ethical Conduct in Publishing

The publishing process is more involved than it may initially seem. There are specific scientific aspects that should be addressed, and, as in so many areas discussed in this book, ethical considerations are paramount. As Piantadosi (2005) noted:

> Reporting the results of a clinical trial is one of the most important aspects of clinical research. Investigators have an obligation to each other, the study participants, and the scientific community to disseminate results in a competent and timely manner (p. 479).

Published journal articles are read by scientists and clinicians, and there is an expectation that the results and interpretations presented are reputable and reliable. Unfortunately, this is not always the case. Like many complex human endeavors, imperfections are not absent. All parties involved in publishing have responsibilities. First, authors have a responsibility to present their research honestly and fully. Two common areas of concern from the reviewers' and readers' perspective are:

- Did the authors leave out information and analyses that did not readily fit in with the desired message of the paper?
- Did the authors present carefully selected *post hoc* analyses as *a priori* planned analyses and make more of their results than they should have?

Reviewers also have a responsibility. Piantadosi (2005) noted that "Limitations of peer review include unqualified, biased, tired, or inattentive reviewers." However, as he also noted, "currently there are no good alternatives for judging the relative merits of scientific papers."

Throughout this book there has been an emphasis on the acquisition of optimum quality data. As well as presenting this optimum quality data to regulatory agencies, it is imperative to present optimum quality data to readers of the clinical literature. It is of the utmost ethical importance that clinical communications are prepared to the highest degree of science and ethics, since clinicians may base the treatment of individual patients on evidence published in clinical communications in their practice of evidence-based medicine (see Section 13.7).

13.6.3 Guidance on Authoring Journal Publications

Guidelines for reporting clinical trials in clinical publications are provided by the Consolidated Standards of Reporting Trials (CONSORT) group (see http://www.consort-statement.org). This group publishes statements that are generally accepted as authoritative: Indeed, as Campbell et al. (2004) noted, many journals now require that submissions conform to the CONSORT Statement, first published in 1996 and revised in 2001. The revised CONSORT statement (see Moher et al., 2001) was entitled "The CONSORT statement: revised recommendations for improving the quality of reports of parallel group randomized trials." Given this book's primary focus on parallel group trials, this guidance is particularly relevant. Given the ease of accessing this statement, readers are recommended to read this statement in its original form.

There is also a CONSORT statement concerning the reporting of cluster randomized trials (recall Section 5.6.2). The added complexities of these studies mean that reporting guidance specifically for these trials is appropriate (see Campbell et al., 2004). Additionally, the CONSORT group has published a statement on reporting equivalence and noninferiority randomized trials (see Piaggio et al., 2006).

13.6.4 Issues Concerning Authorship on a Clinical Communication

An important issue on multiauthored papers is deciding who should be an author (single-authored empirical reports are extremely rare since contemporary clinical research typically requires considerable collaboration). Since many people are involved in the execution of a clinical trial, appropriate criteria are needed to decide on those who will be listed as authors. As in so many instances in this book, both scientific and ethical issues need to be addressed. It is unethical for someone who should not be an author to expect to be so.

Dodson and Abendschein (2005) noted that authors are generally members of the research team who have participated in one or more of the following "tasks":

- Making intellectual contributions to the project.
- Participating in the actual writing of the manuscript.
- Reviewing and approving the final version of the manuscript.

They also observed that "department chairs and division chiefs do not automatically qualify as senior authors."

Piantadosi (2005) commented authoritatively on authorship issues concerning the reporting of clinical trials as follows:

> In the past, it was common for authorship to be a "reward" for contributions to collaborative clinical trials. Physicians placing the most patients on study were often listed as authors of the report, even if they had little or nothing to do with the preparation or editing of the manuscript. This practice is no

> longer satisfactory. Most journal editors require all authors to have contributed substantially to the *report* and to agree with the material that it contains. Authors who do not help with the actual writing of the paper cannot give such assurances (p. 498).

13.6.5 Publication Bias

Piantadosi (2005) defined publication bias as a "tendency for studies with positive results, namely those finding significant differences, to be published in journals in preference to those with negative findings." This is a major concern in that the overall picture painted by the clinical literature on a particular topic can be skewed, or biased.

Bowers et al. (2006) noted that publication bias can arise from various sources, including:

- Journals tend to favor accepting studies showing positive outcomes, i.e., statistically significant differences between treatments, in favor of negative outcomes (as just noted in Piantadosi's definition).
- Studies with positive findings are more likely to be published in English language journals.
- Studies with positive results are more likely to be cited.
- Studies with positive results are more likely to be published in more than one journal. (Publishing results from a study in more than one journal is an ethical issue in itself. While it might be acceptable, even helpful, to publish separate parts of a large study in separate reports, there is a fine line between this and "double publishing").
- Some studies are never submitted for publication. These may include studies which fail to show a positive result and studies that have unfavorable results.

If the typical $p<0.05$ level of statistical significance is adopted by many studies, 1 trial in 20 would be expected to demonstrate a significant effect even if there is no treatment effect. If trials demonstrating positive results are more likely to be published, there is an immediate problem of distortion in the cumulative clinical literature (Matthews, 2006). While changes in certain journal publication practices are leading to some progress in this area, the existing literature will not be affected retrospectively by any future changes.

Publication bias can also influence published literature in an additional way. Two kinds of summary papers, systematic reviews and meta-analyses, bring together many published papers and provide a unifying report. These papers, and the implications of publication bias, are considered in the next section.

13.6.6 Systematic Reviews, Meta-Analyses, and Publication Bias

When reviewing the published literature, it is no small task to find all of the articles that have been published in a specific area of interest. Even when one does a thorough job of locating these articles, their results can be more disparate than one might expect. As Bowers et al. (2006) noted, this disparity can be influenced by several factors, including the employment of highly selected subject samples (which will be different in each case) and smallish sample sizes.

Two kinds of publication can help make sense of a set of differing, and even conflicting, conclusions from a collection of articles on a given topic. One is a systematic review. The strategy in this case is to describe, summarize, and collate the studies in a nonquantitative manner to look for emerging patterns or pictures of evidence. A quantitative approach is provided by the technique of meta-analysis. The results of the different studies are combined according to certain rules, and an overall test statistic is provided. The interpretation of this test statistic leads to the overall "message" of the meta-analysis.

The problem of publication bias can have a profound impact on the messages conveyed by systematic reviews and meta-analyses. When preparing to write these types of papers, authors typically conduct a computer search for articles that meet certain criteria. Examples of these criteria might be:

- Published in an English language journal.
- Published between 1995 and 2006.
- Describes original results from a randomized clinical trial.
- Contains the key words X, Y, and Z.

It was noted in the previous section that studies with positive findings are more likely to be published in English language journals. The first criterion in the bulleted list just presented therefore gives articles with positive findings a better chance of capture in the computer search process and, therefore, inclusion in the systematic review or meta-analysis. The fact that studies with positive results are more likely to be published in more than one journal (noted in the previous section) also gives these articles a better chance of capture in the computer search process and inclusion in the systematic review or meta-analysis.

From a clinical practice perspective, a clinician's treatment of a patient may be influenced by the results of a meta-analysis. Therefore, if the result is influenced by the fact that the articles included in the analysis were not truly representative of all evaluations of the treatment, the result is not likely to be representative either. The issue of publication bias therefore is of critical importance in the context of evidence-based medicine.

13.7 EVIDENCE-BASED MEDICINE

Evidence-based medicine was defined by Sackett et al. (1996) as follows:

> Evidence based medicine is the conscientious, explicit, and judicious use of current best evidence in making decisions about the care of individual patients. The practice of evidence based medicine means integrating individual clinical expertise with the best available external clinical evidence from systematic research. By individual clinical expertise we mean the proficiency and judgment that individual clinicians acquire through clinical experience and clinical practice. Increased expertise is reflected in many ways, but especially in more effective and efficient diagnosis and in the more thoughtful identification and compassionate use of individual patients' predicaments, rights, and preferences in making clinical decisions about their care.

There are two components to evidence-based medicine and two related sets of responsibilities. The first component is clinical research. Clinical research is a scientific endeavor that provides evidence concerning potential therapeutic interventions. This book has focused on one particular therapeutic intervention, drug therapy. Once clinical trials have been conducted, the evidence obtained is published in clinical communications in journals. Everyone involved in clinical research has the responsibility to provide the best possible evidence in this manner. As noted throughout the book, this includes all aspects of clinical research: study design, experimental methodology and clinical operations, analysis and interpretation, and also accurate and complete representation of study findings in clinical communications as discussed in Section 13.6.

The second component of evidence-based medicine is clinical practice (see also Mayer, 2004; Straus et al., 2005). Clinicians have the responsibility of providing the best possible care to each of their individual patients. One part of being able to provide this optimum care is remaining aware of pertinent evidence that is published in clinical communications (as mentioned in the previous section, this is no small task). It is also incumbent on clinicians to be able to decide for themselves if the evidence presented in a clinical communication is good evidence and if the message of a systematic review or a meta-analysis is justified based on the quality of the report. As Katz (2001) commented:

> Part of the burden for the responsible cultivation of higher standards and better outcomes in medicine falls, naturally, to researchers and those who screen and publish their findings. But application is ultimately the responsibility of the clinician,

> who is obligated to consider not only the pertinence of particular evidence to his or her practice but the adequacy and reliability of the evidence itself (p. xvi).

Therefore, an appreciation of study design, experimental methodology, statistical analysis, and clinical interpretation is vital for clinicians who must decide whether the evidence presented in clinical communications is adequate and reliable and therefore an appropriate basis for clinical care. Clinicians, clinical research professionals, and students engaged in clinical writing are encouraged to use Bowers et al.'s (2006) book *Understanding Clinical Papers*, not only as a guide to understanding clinical papers but also as a guide to writing clinical papers in a manner that is readily understood.

13.7.1 Scientific Evidence and Clinical Judgment

In addition to remaining abreast of clinical communications and evaluating the scientific validity of their results and interpretations, a clinician also has to use clinical judgment in providing clinical care. As we have noted, the evidence from a clinical trial is not perfectly generalizable to the target population with the disease or condition of interest. Therefore, a clinician is constantly faced with the task of deciding to what extent the information from a given clinical trial applies to a particular patient. As Katz (2001) observed:

> If our patient is older than, younger than, sicker than, healthier than, ethnically different from, taller, shorter, simply different from the subjects of a study, do the results pertain?...No degree of evidence will fully chart the expanse of idiosyncrasy in human health and disease. Thus, to work skillfully with evidence is to acknowledge its limits. All of the art and all of the science of medicine depends on how artfully and scientifically we as practitioners reach our decisions. The art of clinical decision making is judgment, an even more difficult concept to grapple with than evidence (pp. xi, xvii).

Decision making and the role of judgment are discussed further in Section 14.5.

Part V

Integrative Discussion

14

Unifying Themes and Concluding Comments

14.1 Introduction

This book has provided an introductory overview of the immensely complex process of new drug development. Since various aspects of this process have been discussed individually in the preceding chapters, this final chapter takes a more global view. It brings together threads that have run throughout the individual chapters and presents an integrative summary of topics discussed to date. It also discusses pharmacogenetics, pharmacogenomics, and pharmacoproteomics, topics of interest to many scientists, pharmaceutical and biopharmaceutical companies, and clinicians at this time. These discussions build upon material that has been covered in several chapters.

14.2 Ethical Considerations

Looking back across the previous chapters' discussion of new drug development, several themes emerge:

- It requires that attention be paid to ethical considerations.
- It requires that attention be paid to design, methodological, and analytical considerations.
- Pharmacokinetic and pharmacodynamic considerations are of interest at every stage of the process.
- Many decisions have to be made throughout the process, and each has major consequences.
- There is much more subjectivity in this decision making than might be initially thought.
- The ultimate goal is to change patients' biology for the better.

This section addresses ethical considerations, and then the other items in this list are discussed in turn.

Ethical considerations are pervasive throughout new drug development. The need for ethical treatment of all subjects who are willing to participate in clinical research—an activity that is designed for the greater good, not for their individual benefit—is paramount. Also, since it is unethical to include subjects in a study where poor design and/or poor methodology leads to less-than-optimum data and therefore less-than-optimum answers to the study's research question, everyone involved in clinical research has the responsibility to act in an ethical manner. Just like Statistics, ethics are not simply something for "someone else" to worry about.

New Drug Development: Design, Methodology, and Analysis. By J. Rick Turner

In the previous chapters, discussions of ethical considerations have occurred in many contexts, including:

- Designing a study in an ethical manner such that the design is capable of producing optimum quality data.
- Subject recruitment, including providing informed consent.
- Sample-size estimation. A study design requires sufficient subjects but not an unnecessarily large subject sample.
- Conducting all aspects of a study in the best manner possible such that the methodology is capable of producing optimum quality data.
- Data monitoring committees face difficult ethical challenges, in particular deciding whether a clinical trial should be terminated early.
- Authors have an ethical responsibility to report information accurately and fully in clinical communications, since these directly impact patient care.

As noted in Section 1.8.1, Derenzo and Moss (2006) captured these sentiments very well:

> Each study component has an ethical aspect. The ethical aspects of a clinical trial cannot be separated from the scientific objectives. Segregation of ethical issues from the full range of study design components demonstrates a flaw in understanding the fundamental nature of research involving human subjects. Compartmentalization of ethical issues is inconsistent with a well-run trial. Ethical and scientific considerations are intertwined (p. 4).

14.3 DESIGN, METHODOLOGY, AND ANALYSIS

Given the statements in Chapter 1 that design, methodology, and analysis are central characters in this book, it is not surprising that they have been frequently encountered throughout the previous chapters. It has been noted that design, methodology, and analysis are of importance across the entire spectrum of new drug development, including drug discovery and design, nonclinical research, clinical development, and postmarketing surveillance. A vast array of numerical information is collected and analyzed during these various stages of research.

In nonclinical research, attention to detail is every bit as important as in clinical development. As Gad (2006) observed, "the importance of nonclinical laboratory studies demands that they be conducted according to scientifically sound protocols and with meticulous attention to quality."

Early-phase clinical studies involve relatively small numbers of subjects. However, this does not mean that design, methodology, and analysis are any less critical. Machin and Campbell (2005) noted that these early-phase clinical studies provide key information for the drug development process and that it is "essential that they are carefully designed, painstakingly conducted, and meticulously reported in full."

While the nature of the analyses of data from therapeutic confirmatory clinical trials is relatively straightforward compared with those undertaken in earlier stages of clinical development, supreme care should again be taken in all aspects of design, methodology, and analysis, since only then can optimum quality data be used to provide optimum answers to well-constructed research questions. Chapter 10 noted that safety data are typically presented descriptively at this time but that this may change in due course. By the time that therapeutic confirmatory trials are conducted, there should be a small number of precisely asked research questions that address the efficacy of the drug.

In a fixed design trial, the analyses used to provide compelling evidence of efficacy are typically straightforward: They may be somewhat more sophisticated in group sequential studies and adaptive design trials. As emphasized throughout the book, however, while statistical evidence of efficacy is required by regulatory agencies at this time, the clinical significance of the treatment effect is ultimately the primary concern. By the time that therapeutic confirmatory trials are conducted, the sponsor will have a good idea of the drug's efficacy from earlier clinical studies. These later trials will only be conducted if they are likely to confirm that the treatment effect is indeed clinically significant.

14.3.1 Reducing Bias and Improving Precision

Statistical methodology has two important goals: reducing bias (see Evanoff, 2005) and improving precision. The process of randomization, as does the procedure of blinding, reduces bias (the word "reduces" is deliberately used here, since total elimination is not a feasible goal). Statistical inferences are based on the use of randomization to reduce bias to the greatest extent possible and ensure comparability of the treatment groups with respect to pertinent variables such as age, gender, and other important prognostic factors (Chow and Liu, 2004). Analysis of covariance can also be used in this context to address influences that could not be addressed by randomization (recall Section 11.4.2).

Improving precision as much as possible is also a highly desirable attribute in a study design, and statistical methodology aims to improve precision in several ways, including reducing error variance. Better measurements will yield data that provide a more precise answer, e.g., narrower confidence intervals around the treatment effect obtained in a trial.

14.3.2 Our Operational Definition of Statistics Revisited

This book's operational definition of Statistics was presented in Section 1.3. According to this definition, Statistics can be thought of as an integrated discipline that is important in all of the following activities:

- Identifying a research question that needs to be answered.
- Deciding upon the design of the study, the methodology that will be employed, and the numerical information (data) that will be collected.
- Presenting the design, methodology, and data to be collected in a study protocol. This study protocol specifies the manner of data collection, and addresses all methodological considerations necessary to ensure the collection of optimum quality data for subsequent statistical analysis.
- Identifying the statistical techniques that will be used to describe and analyze the data in an associated statistical analysis plan, which should be written in conjunction with the study protocol.
- Describing and analyzing the data. This includes analyzing the variation in the data to see if there is compelling evidence that the drug is safe and effective. This process includes evaluation of the statistical significance of the results obtained and, very importantly, their clinical significance.
- Presenting the results of a clinical study to a regulatory agency in a clinical study report and presenting the results to the clinical community in journal publications.

This operational definition of Statistics may have seemed rather expansive when it was first encountered in Chapter 1. In this concluding chapter, I hope it may seem much more appropriate. As has been noted many times, statistical awareness is essential throughout the entire drug development process, from designing a study to answer a research question right through to presenting the study results to regulatory agencies and the clinical community.

14.3.3 Numerical Representations of Biological Information

The data acquired in a clinical trial are not simply numbers: They are numerical representations of biologically important information. The number 9 is meaningful by itself (it is an integer between 8 and 10). However, in a clinical database, the digit 9 may represent a decrease of 9 mmHg seen in a subject's SBP following the administration of an investigational antihypertensive drug for several weeks. In this context, the digit 9 is a numerical representation of biologically important information concerning a change in blood pressure. The employment of the discipline of Statistics is a means to an end here, and the end is producing a drug that is safe and has a beneficial therapeutic effect on a patient's biological well-being.

In this context, drugs prescribed in psychiatric care are considered to have a beneficial therapeutic effect on a patient's biological well-being. While some sources differentiate between psychological well-being and physical well-being, and therapies such as cognitive behavioral therapy may also be used in psychological and psychiatric counseling, pharmacological agents exert their influence via biological changes that contribute to the patient's well-being.

14.3.4 Some Thoughts on the *p*-Value

The requirement to show statistical significance in therapeutic confirmatory trials places a certain importance on *a priori* hypothesis testing. However, as we have seen, there is much more to clinical research than *p*-values. Piantadosi (2005) commented on this issue as follows:

> There are many circumstances in which *p*-values are useful, particularly for hypothesis tests specified *a priori*. However, they have properties that make them poor summaries of clinical effects. In particular, they do not convey the magnitude of a clinical effect. The size of the *p*-value is a consequence of two things: the magnitude of the estimated treatment difference and its estimated variability (which is itself a consequence of sample size). Thus the *p*-value partially reflects the size of the experiment, which has no biological importance. The *p*-value also hides the size of the treatment, which does have major biological importance.

Piantadosi (2005) also addressed a commonly expressed view when a researcher obtains a nonsignificant result in a study. It is often said that the estimated treatment effect obtained might be statistically significant in a larger sample. This statement is a true statement, but not a helpful one. It is true because any non-zero effect will attain statistical significance in a large enough sample. What would be helpful instead would be to focus on the size of the estimated treatment effect and its clinical (biological) significance. It is very useful to remember that *p*-values "incompletely characterize the biologically important effects in the data" (Piantadosi, 2005; see also Blume and Peipert, 2003).

14.3.5 The Use of Confidence Intervals

Confidence intervals are extremely informative in clinical research since they do focus on the estimated treatment effect and therefore facilitate consideration of its clinical significance. As Fletcher and Fletcher (2005) noted succinctly and powerfully, confidence intervals "put the emphasis where it belongs, on the size of the effect." The width of a confidence interval around an experimentally determined treatment effect, and hence the range of plausible values for the population treatment effect, provides very important information about the clinical significance of the treatment.

As we saw in Chapter 8, confidence intervals can be used to deduce levels of statistical significance: While they do not yield precise *p*-values, they reveal whether or not a given level of statistical significance is achieved. More importantly, they are uniquely informative in assessing clinical significance. Therefore, confidence intervals offer a tremendous advantage over *p*-values in the clinical context, and they are extremely important in drug development. They have become an important way of reporting the main results in clinical research (Fletcher and Fletcher, 2005).

14.4 PHARMACOKINETICS AND PHARMACODYNAMICS

Pharmacokinetic and pharmacodynamic considerations have been discussed several times in the book. It was noted in the Preface that there would be a certain degree of planned repetition in the book: Concepts are introduced at one point and then integrated with other material at a later point. This has been true for pharmacokinetics and pharmacodynamics. It is also true for some of the genetic discussions that follow in this chapter.

An investigational drug's pharmacokinetic/pharmacodynamic profile is of critical importance in determining its therapeutic usefulness, and assessment of this profile continues throughout the entire spectrum of new drug development. Pharmacokinetic issues are a major factor in a drug's success after it has received marketing approval. A drug product certainly has to be safe and effective, but it also has to be convenient to use if it is going to be widely used and commercially successful. Pharmacokinetic characteristics are a major determinant of how convenient a drug is to use.

Pharmacokinetic issues are being increasingly addressed in drug discovery. If a drug candidate has a pharmacokinetic profile that suggests potential later problems, it is better that the drug fails earlier in the discovery/development process rather than later. If the drug candidate looks promising, its pharmacokinetic profile will be evaluated in nonclinical studies. If this looks promising, the pharmacokinetic profile of the investigational drug will be evaluated in human pharmacology clinical studies. One of the most common reasons for not continuing with clinical development of a drug is an unsuitable pharmacokinetic profile, and it is therefore strategically important to evaluate a drug's pharmacokinetic profile in early-phase drug development.

The extensive study of the pharmacodynamic (and toxicodynamic) potential and properties of a drug is also of interest throughout the entire development process. Maximizing interactions between the drug and its target receptor (and minimizing interactions between the drug and nontarget receptors) is of considerable interest in drug discovery and design. The biological signal that results from the energetic interaction between the drug and the target receptor has a beneficial effect on biological systems. Therapeutic exploratory and therapeutic confirmatory clinical trials address the topic of the drug's efficacy more formally.

14.5 DECISION MAKING

If forced to summarize the purposes of study design, experimental methodology, and statistical analysis in one sentence each, the following might be suitable:

- Study design: Determining the best (practical) way of collecting accurate data, i.e., unbiased numerical representations of biologically important information.
- Experimental methodology: Acquiring optimum quality data.
- Statistical analysis: Describing, summarizing, analyzing, and interpreting the data collected to answer the study's research question.

Expanding on the last point, numerical representations of biologically important information facilitate answers to questions that arise during the process of new drug development and thus provide the basis for making the best possible decision at that time given the best evidence available at that time. (It is quite appropriate to use later additional information to come to a new decision.)

Many decisions during the process of new drug development concern whether or not to proceed to the next step in the process. Adequate evidence needs to be obtained, and documented, to permit careful consideration of the benefits and risks of proceeding. Given a finite amount of resources and, particularly in the case of larger pharmaceutical companies, a choice of drug candidates upon which to focus these resources, it is financially prudent to proceed only if there is a reasonable chance of success (the definition of "reasonable" being unique to each sponsor and drug candidate). As Wurst and Guernsey (2006) commented, "If a compound fails to meet expectations, the project should be terminated, and the earlier a candidate is eliminated from development, the fewer penalties the company pays in investment and opportunity costs." While business driven, the choice to pursue development programs that are likely to yield successful drugs is arguably in the best interests of patients: Pursuing development plans for drug candidates that are likely to fail reduces the sponsor's ability to work on drugs that may get approved and help patients.

14.5.1 The Subjective Nature of Many Decisions

The title of this section may be surprising at first. The process of science, one may think, produces clear-cut answers, and scientists pride themselves on the objectivity inherent in their disciplines and, accordingly, on conducting business in an objective manner. Clinical science, clinical research, and clinical practice, however, require a combination of objective information and informed judgment. Since all judgment is subjective, subjectivity is an integral part of clinical science, clinical research, and clinical practice.

In this context, the word "subjective" does not carry the potentially negative connotations that may accompany it in other realms. All of us would likely welcome the medical opinion of a very experienced and well-informed clinician when making a decision concerning several possible therapeutic regimens. The opinion offered would be the clinician's best clinical judgment based on the best available evidence at that time. In the context of study design, Piantadosi (2005) made the following comment:

> It is a mistake not to recognize the subjectivity that is present, or to design and interpret studies in formulaic ways. We could more appropriately view experimental designs as devices that encapsulate both objective plans along with unavoidable subjectivity (p.131).

Consider two examples from previous chapters that illustrate this. In Chapter 9, discussions of sample-size estimation emphasized that the process is indeed one of estimation rather than pure calculation. A calculation is certainly executed, but the values that are placed into the appropriate formula are chosen by the sponsor. On each occasion, the sponsor must consider the influences of the choices that are made and make the most appropriate decision in the specific context of that trial. In Chapter 11, equivalence and noninferiority designs were discussed. In addition to the calculations that are involved using the data collected in a trial, equivalence or noninferiority margins must be established before the trial commences. Their choice is a clinical choice, not a statistical choice, and subjectivity is necessarily involved in this choice. Thus, the discipline of Statistics certainly involves using informed judgments. Statistics really is an art as well as a science, a sentiment well expressed by Katz (2001) as cited in Chapter 13.

Consider also the decisions that must be made by regulatory agencies. From many perspectives, the role of regulatory agencies is far from easy. For example, they have to decide if it is "appropriate" to allow a sponsor to commence clinical testing based on data submitted in an IND. It has been noted several times that no animal model is a perfect predictor of human responses to an investigational drug, and so the decision to allow a sponsor to commence clinical trials requires a judgment call. An enormous amount of information has to be provided to regulatory agencies to allow them to make this decision, but it is still a judgment call, albeit a very well informed judgment.

The same is true when a regulatory agency evaluates the evidence presented in an NDA or BLA. Again, a tremendous amount of information is presented following the conduct of clinical trials, but these data cannot guarantee that serious adverse drug reactions will not be seen once the drug is approved and taken by a large number of patients. The agency has to evaluate all of the data in the marketing application and consider the benefit/risk ratio of approving the drug. This is a tremendous responsibility. Therefore, as noted in Chapter 13, while the randomized controlled trials that we have discussed in this book remain the gold standard for evaluating the efficacy of a new drug in preapproval clinical trials, and they do provide (some) safety data, they cannot be regarded as the sole source of safety data or as a guaranteed predictor of the drug's effectiveness in the target population. In a real sense, marketing approval of a new drug can be regarded as the beginning of its true evaluation.

14.6 PHARMACOGENETICS

Pharmacogenetics studies the contribution of genetic variation to the variation in response to pharmacotherapy. Interest lies both with desired therapeutic effects and with the range and severity of adverse events. When a given drug is administered to different patients for whom, based on the best available diagnostic evidence, it is appropriate, many of them will safely experience a therapeutic benefit. However, there are other possible outcomes that may be experienced by a relatively small number of patients:

- Individuals may not show a beneficial therapeutic response (non-responders).
- Individuals may show an undesired excessive therapeutic response (e.g., becoming hypotensive instead of normotensive following the administration of an antihypertensive agent).
- Individuals may show relatively serious undesired effects (adverse responders).

While other factors (e.g., existing disease, concomitant medication, nutrition, and use of tobacco and alcohol) can influence why different people respond differently to a given drug, the predominant factor is genetic variation, specifically variation in the structure of the target receptor and in pharmacokinetics (Primrose and Twyman, 2006).

We have discussed both target receptors and pharmacokinetics in this book. Protein manufacture is under direct genetic control, and two factors are of particular relevance here. First, the precise structure and function of protein macromolecules (receptors) targeted by a specific drug molecule will vary in different individuals. Since the structure and function of the protein are directly related to how the drug molecule will interact with that protein, individuals' responses to the drug will vary. Second, there are genetic variations in metabolic enzymes (proteins) and hence metabolism. Both of these processes fall neatly into the domain of pharmacoproteomics (see Section 14.8).

The diversity in drug effects among different individuals presents a major problem in clinical medicine and drug development. Most approved drugs are not effective for all patients; additionally, drugs can be very toxic, even fatal, for some patients (Meyer, 2002). Interactions occur between an individual's genetic information that codes for pharmacodynamic and pharmacokinetic determinants of a drug's effects and environmental factors. The resulting expression, lack of expression, or over-expression of certain genes influences the drug effects experienced by individuals. As noted, these effects include lack of drug efficacy and drug toxicity.

14.6.1 Genetic Variation in Metabolism, Pharmacokinetics, and Pharmacodynamics

Ferkol et al. (2005) listed three major mechanisms by which genetic variation can produce variation in individual responses to drugs:

- Variation within the drug target (e.g., ion channels). This may lead to altered drug efficacy and differences in the expression of a physiological phenotype.
- Variation associated with altered distribution, metabolism, or uptake of the drug. This may lead to enhanced drug clearance, impaired drug clearance, or inactivation of the drug.
- Variation resulting in an unintended drug action.

Proteins are biological products of an individual's genetic information, and proteins commonly function as drug receptors. This provides a direct molecular genetic link to discussions of why some people react to a drug very differently from the majority of patients who receive it. Since the pharmacodynamic effect of a drug is the result of the interaction between the drug and the receptor, genetically determined individual differences in drug receptor structure may lead to individual differences in response to a drug (both therapeutic and toxic).

Additionally, metabolic pathways are also biological products of an individual's genetic information. The genome-transcriptome-proteome information flow, a more contemporary expression of the "DNA-to-RNA-to-proteins" information flow noted in Chapter 3, facilitates the creation of the metabolic pathways that comprise the metabolic system and, therefore, facilitates the creation of the resulting organism. As noted earlier in the book, at the time of writing, a reasonable estimate of the number of human genes is 25,000–30,000. It is also reasonable to estimate that these genes facilitate the production of more than a million proteins and these proteins interact in a complex manner to create hundreds of millions of metabolic pathways, the metabolic basis of life (Augen, 2005).

This enormous array of metabolic pathways leads to the uniqueness of individuals. In a real biological sense, each person's individuality is the result of, and can be represented by, their individual and unique set of metabolic pathways (Augen, 2005). Given that pharmacokinetic activity is a key determinant of how well a drug is able to exert its pharmacodynamic effect (or how good a chance it gets to do so), and given that metabolism is a key determinant of pharmacokinetic activity, genetic influence on metabolism may lead to individual differences in response to a drug. As Kalow (2005) noted, "Pharmacogenetics is still largely considered a story of person-to-person differences in drug metabolism and response."

14.7 PHARMACOGENOMICS

Genotype information, information about a person's whole genetic make-up, permits the possibility of pharmacological therapy targeted at particular individuals based on this knowledge. The field of pharmacogenomics involves the use of genomic technologies in assessing differential responses to drugs. The terms "pharmacogenomics" (PGx) and "pharmacogenetics" are not synonymous. Rather, thanks to molecular genetics and genomics, the term pharmacogenomics "reflects the evolution of pharmacogenetics into the study of the entire spectrum of genes that determine drug response, including the assessment of the diversity of the human genome and its clinical consequences" (Meyer, 2002). As Rothstein (2003) noted, pharmacogenetics addresses "the role of genetic variation in differential response to pharmaceuticals" and pharmacogenomics addresses "the use of genomic technologies in assessing differential response to pharmaceuticals."

Over the last few years, pharmacogenomic studies have become an increasingly greater part of drug development. As Lesko and Woodcock (2005) noted:

> Drug companies reportedly collect DNA samples from subjects in approximately 80% of clinical studies so that they can have the chance to identify genomic biomarkers of drug safety, efficacy, and dosing. The promise of PGx lies in its potential to identify sources of interindividual variability in drug response (both efficacy and safety) that arise from genomic differences in disease pathophysiology and/or genomic differences in drug pharmacology (p. 273).

These authors also noted that the FDA "has become a proactive and thoughtful advocate of PGx" and that it believes it has a responsibility as a public health agency to play "a leading role in bringing about the translation of PGx, as well as other emerging technologies, from bench to bedside to facilitate drug development and improve the benefit/risk of drug treatments in the marketplace" (Lesko and Woodcock, 2005). See also Brown (2003), Deverka and Magnus (2005), Lesko et al. (2006), and Roses (2004) for further discussion.

14.7.1 Precision Medicine

The practice of precision medicine is predicated on knowledge of a person's genotype. The term "precision medicine" is deliberately used here instead of other common terms such as personalized medicine and individualized medicine: Clinicians, as they will argue forcefully and very reasonably, have always practiced personalized medicine to the limit of current knowledge. Thoughtful clinical care of a patient has always involved, and always will involve, using all available evidence concerning an individual patient's unique set of circumstances and knowledge of all available treatment options to tailor a course of treatment accordingly. The major difference in the context of present discussions is that, in the future, clinicians will likely have access to detailed information about the biological make-up of individual patients under their care. As Monkhouse (2006b) commented:

> Pharmacogenomic studies promise to revolutionize medicine by providing clinicians with prospective knowledge regarding the likelihood of an individual patient's response to a particular medication and, ultimately, the identification of patients who might benefit from targeted dosing of the drug or alternate drug therapy (pp. 26-27).

14.8 PHARMACOPROTEOMICS: PROTEOMICS AND DRUG THERAPY

The FDA recently released its Critical Path Opportunities List (see Section 14.10). One of six broad topic areas of opportunity listed is "Harnessing Bioinformatics." Accordingly, the field of bioinformatics, which was introduced in Section 3.4, is discussed here in more detail. Given the importance of drug receptors throughout the book and the fact that drug receptors are typically proteins, the contribution of bioinformatics to our knowledge of proteins is of particular interest here. As Holmes et al. (2005) commented:

> Although much attention has been paid to the sequencing aspects of genome projects, the eventual end goal of these projects actually is to determine how the genome builds life through proteins. DNA has been the focus of attention because the tools for studying it are more advanced and because it is at the heart of the cell, carrying all the information—the blueprint—for life. However, a blueprint without a builder is not very useful, and the proteins are the primary builders within the cell (p. 446).

Soloviev et al. (2004) captured the nature of the developing field of proteomics in the following:

> Characterization of the complement of expressed proteins from a single genome is a central focus of the evolving field of proteomics. Monitoring the expression and properties of a large number of proteins provides important information about the

> physiological state of a cell and an organism. A cell can express a large number of different proteins and the expression profile (the number of proteins expressed and the expression levels) vary in different cell types, explaining why different cells perform different functions (p. 218).

Proteomics involves the systematic analysis of proteins to determine their identity, quantity, and function (Soloviev et al., 2004). Until recently, the study of proteins focused on individual proteins using various established techniques such as gel-electrophoresis and chromatography. The advent of high-throughput automated technologies is now facilitating the move toward simultaneous analysis of all the proteins in a defined protein population (Soloviev et al., 2004, see also Jones and Warren, 2006).

14.8.1 Studying Proteins

One of the major facilitators of DNA research has been researchers' ability to generate almost unlimited quantities (copies) of a target nucleic acid sequence by using polymerase chain reaction (PCR) techniques. Currently, however, there is not an equivalent technique for proteins, and so research techniques have to study the very small amount of molecules that are produced *in vivo*. Three strategies of interest in protein research are:

- Structural studies: X-ray crystallography and nuclear magnetic resonance spectroscopy are discussed shortly.
- Functional studies: Mass spectroscopy, discussed shortly, can be used to examine "the regulation, timing, and location of protein expression" (Holmes et al., 2005).
- Interaction studies: These studies are interested in interactions between proteins with other molecules in a cell and also protein-protein interactions; these interactions result in the cell's molecular machinery (see Hudes et al., 2004, Loregian and Palu, 2005).

14.8.2 The Proteome

The 25,000–30,000 genes in humans comprise the human genome. However, the number of proteins in the proteome is considerably larger: A value on the order of one million was noted in Section 14.6.1. This phenomenon is the result of "the simple although not widely appreciated fact that multiple, distinct proteins can result from one gene" (Holmes et al., 2005).

The journey from genome to proteome is not a straightforward one. Holmes et al. (2005) represented this journey in a multistep process, starting with a gene of interest in the genome:

- DNA replication results in many gene forms.
- RNA transcription leads to pre-messenger RNA.
- RNA maturation results in mature messenger RNA.
- Protein translation results in an immature protein.
- Protein maturation results in a mature protein in the proteome (post-translational modifications are possible here).

The tremendous diversity of proteins in the proteome is facilitated by multiple possible means of protein expression. At each stage in the multistep process just described, alternative mechanisms produce variants of the "standard" product. The combination of possible variations in the multistep process results in an enormous potential diversity in the resulting proteome (Holmes et al., 2005).

14.8.3 Very Large Numbers and Very Small Numbers

The human brain is not very good at dealing with very large numbers or very small numbers. Throughout the vast majority of history, humans dealt with moderate numbers that represented how many people lived in a village, how much food needed to be collected to feed them, and how many days it took to walk, run, or ride to another settlement. The number of calculations that a present-day supercomputer can perform in a second (a very large number) and the scales of measurement in nanotechnology (very small numbers) are very recent additions to the scope of human interests. So too are the molecular structures of DNA, RNA, and proteins. DNA molecules are comprised of a very large number of atoms. The other end of the spectrum of sizes is well exemplified by electron dynamics. Ultrafast electron flow in a biochemical reaction is measured in attoseconds (10^{-18} sec), i.e., in quintillionths of a second. At this point, further quantification and illustration of very large numbers and very small numbers are not really necessary: It is sufficient to say that bioinformatics utilizes systems that can analyze a very large amount of information about some very small particles of material.

14.8.4 Bioinformatics and Pharmacoproteomics

An organism's genome is the collection of all genes within that organism. Sequencing genomes is far from easy, but it is easier than compiling an organism's putative proteome, the collection of all the proteins produced by the organism's genes. While genomics is of great interest in certain aspects of pharmaceutical therapy, in particular pharmacogenomics, proteomics is of pervasive interest in drug therapeutics since so many drug receptors for both small-molecule and macromolecule drugs are proteins. This leads to the domain of pharmacoproteomics.

Bioinformatics is of enormous benefit in proteomic and pharmacoproteomic research. Structural bioinformatics and functional bioinformatics are powerful allies in deciphering the information coded in a protein's primary sequence of amino acid residues and thus predicting, or modeling, the protein's structure and function. Since so many drug receptors are proteins, greater knowledge of the structure of the proteins will improve our ability to discover/design drug candidates that may interact with these receptors in a beneficial therapeutic manner.

There are 20 naturally occurring amino acids. Proteins are thus written in a 20-letter language of amino acid residues (Ofran and Rost, 2005), and the function of each protein is encrypted in its amino acid sequence. However, as these authors noted:

> Although it is rather simple to determine protein sequences experimentally, it remains quite difficult (and sometimes even impossible) to determine protein structure and function experimentally (p. 198).

We will first look briefly at two experimental techniques used in attempts to determine protein structure experimentally and then discuss computational or prediction strategies for protein structure and function.

14.8.5 X-Ray Crystallography

As the name implies, this technique uses both X-rays and crystals. Small protein crystals are exposed to a beam of X-rays, whose wavelength is approximately the size of an atom. The X-rays are diffracted by the atoms in the crystal and the diffraction pattern is recorded. While there will be trillions of individual protein molecules in the crystal, this pattern can be analyzed by a computer to reveal the three-dimensional coordinates of key atoms in a stylized "average protein."

While the technique of X-ray crystallography is a complex instrumental and computational procedure, it can reveal the structure of very large macromolecules, which means that it permits the determination of the structure of both cytoplasmic proteins and membrane-bound proteins (proteins that are typically drug targets). While X-ray crystallography is very useful, however, it should be emphasized that proteins studied in this manner are in a crystalline state, a state that does not resemble "the normal physiological (liquid) environment of the cell or body" (Wishart, 2005).

14.8.6 Nuclear Magnetic Resonance Spectroscopy

Nuclear magnetic resonance (NMR) spectroscopy is a considerably newer technique than X-ray crystallography, and it has certain comparative advantages. First, it does not require proteins to be in crystalline form: Proteins can be studied in near-physiological environmental conditions. Second, it is a quicker process. On the other hand, it also has comparative disadvantages. It is limited by the size of the molecule and by the solubility of the molecule being studied, which means that membrane proteins cannot be studied. Also, NMR structures are less precise than X-ray structures, although it should be noted that X-ray structures are typically not perfect either (Wishart, 2005).

14.8.7 Mass Spectroscopy

Mass spectroscopy (MS) is allowing researchers to "map" cellular metabolism to a further extent and, importantly, to "see" many regulatory, or cell signaling, networks for the first time. Cell signaling network mapping is of particular interest because of its role in studying diseases such as cancer, diabetes, and Alzheimer's disease. As Bader and Enright (2005) noted, "A molecule's interacting and reacting partners define its function in a biological system." Biomolecular interaction and pathway analysis falls within the field of bioinformatics. Signaling pathways involve many direct protein-protein relationships and can be mapped using protein-protein interaction detection methods (see Loregian and Palu, 2005).

14.8.8 Predicting Solvent Accessibility

As well as predicting protein structure, it is also of interest to try to predict solvent accessibility from the protein's primary sequence of amino acid residues. Solvent accessibility concerns the area of a protein's surface that is exposed to the surrounding solvent. The importance of this concept is that these accessible regions have the potential to interact with other entities, including endogenous proteins and drugs. Similarly, if the protein of interest is an enzyme, only residues with solvent accessibility could be part of the enzyme's active site. This means that an interaction site of interest, one involved in signal transduction (see Krauss, 2003), requires "spatial accessibility" to the solvent (Ofran and Rost, 2005).

It is important to note that this concept does not negate the importance of other residues that are "land-locked" in the interior of a protein structure—these may play important roles in stabilizing the structure, thereby ensuring that the active site is indeed presented appropriately—but they will not be part of an active site.

Communication between a cell and other cells in its surroundings is based almost exclusively on proteins that are embedded in the cell's membrane. Many proteins pass through the cellular membrane and can therefore interact with molecules on the intracellular side of the membrane as well as with molecules on the extracellular side. These "transmembrane proteins" and their molecular mechanisms are of particular interest in biomedicine (Ofran and Rost, 2005). It is particularly difficult to decipher the structure of transmembrane segments (helices) of proteins experimentally, which makes *in silico* prediction particularly valuable.

14.8.9 *In Silico* Structure and Function Prediction

In silico modeling was introduced in Chapter 3. *In silico* efforts to glean biologically important information about a protein's structure and activity (function) from its amino acid residue sequence have been intense in the last several decades. It is of particular interest to predict several aspects of proteins that we have mentioned:

- Secondary structure.
- Solvent accessibility.
- Transmembrane helices.
- Tertiary structure.

Tremendous amounts of information from the experimental methods of X-ray crystallography and (NMR) spectroscopy and from *in silico* modeling have been entered into databases, and this information is shared by many researchers worldwide. Once the amino acid residue sequence of a new protein of interest has been identified, it is intuitively of interest to search these databases for well-characterized proteins with similar sequences, to note their function, and to consider the possibility that the function of the new protein may be similar. Unfortunately, things are seldom that simple in this field. Proteins with similar primary sequences may have quite different structures and functions, and, taking this one step further, some proteins, termed moonlighting proteins, display different functions depending on their immediate cellular surroundings (Ofran and Rost, 2005).

14.8.10 Predicting Tertiary Structure

While still far from perfect, *in silico* methods of predicting secondary structure and solvent accessibility using only a protein's primary sequence have matured considerably in recent years (Ofran and Rost, 2005). Ability to predict tertiary structure is currently less well developed but improving.

Many of the first bioinformatics programs written were created with the goal of solving the "protein folding problem," i.e., predicting the three-dimensional structure of a protein using only a protein's primary sequence (predicting structure is a necessary forerunner of predicting biological function). Progress is being made in this amazingly difficult and computationally intense field. There are various methods of predicting three-dimensional protein structures (Wishart, 2005):

- Homology (comparative) modeling. This is currently the most powerful and accurate of the three methods. Homologous features are those in different individuals that are descended genetically from the same feature in a common ancestor. Homology modeling predicts the tertiary structure of a protein by using information in a database about an existing homologous protein as a template.
- Threading (fold recognition). This method suggests broad possibilities by attempting to recognize a common fold in proteins that are not homologous.
- *Ab initio* ("predicting from the beginning") methods. This method is aimed at identifying folds for which there is a complete lack of sequence

similarity to existing structures. Currently, it is the least developed method, but it is improving.

High-quality structural models can reveal an enormous amount of biologically important information concerning the function of a protein, how it is related to other proteins, and to what receptor region a drug molecule may or may not bind. As discussed in Chapter 3, this information is very helpful in designing new drugs.

14.8.11 Network-Related Databases and Modeling Pathways

While it is important and informative to create individual databases, the complexity of modeling pathways requires that individual databases be integrated or networked. Bader and Enright (2005) asked the question "What would we want to know from an ideal cell biological experiment?" and then provided their answer:

> The answer is no less than everything: what molecules are in the cell at what time and at what place, how many molecules are there, what molecules they interact with, and the specifics of their interaction dynamics. Ideally, one would want this information not only over the course of the cell cycle, but also in all important environmental conditions and under all known disease states (pp. 254-255).

Biologists have not only "organized" the cell into pathways and modules but also classified these pathways into various types. Each of the main types has a different computational representation in pathway databases. Bader and Enright (2005) discussed three biochemical- and biophysical-based pathways that are modeled:

- Gene regulation pathways. Gene regulation networks involve transcription factors that can activate or repress the expression of a set of genes.
- Metabolic pathways. These involve a series of chemical actions undertaken to change one type of molecule into another.
- Signal transduction (cell signaling) pathways. These pathways are typically defined by binding events, often protein-protein interactions, for the purpose of communicating information from one part of the cell to another.

Captured within the last of these bullet points is the essence of drug therapy: The goal is to administer a drug that will bind with a receptor and lead to a beneficial cascade of biological information flow that produces the desired therapeutic effect.

14.9 THE COSTS OF PHARMACEUTICAL DEVELOPMENT

As Rawlins (2004) commented:

> Humankind has reaped extraordinary benefits from the pharmacological revolution of the twentieth century. Conditions such as poliomyelitis, diphtheria and whooping cough have been largely eliminated in developed countries by immunization. Many lethal communicable diseases can be readily cured with antimicrobial agents. And drugs have improved the quality of life for many people with chronic diseases to an extent that would have been unthinkable in the nineteenth century (p. 360).

However, as he points out, this is no time to rest on our laurels: There are massive unmet medical needs in both developing and developed countries. For example, effective vaccines are needed for HIV/AIDS, malaria, and tuberculosis, and neurodegenerative disorders such as Parkinson's disease and Alzheimer's disease are relatively poorly serviced by current pharmacological therapy.

In this context, there is both very good news and very bad news. Advances in various areas discussed in this book (e.g., bioinformatics, combinatorial chemistry, high-throughput screening, molecular biology and molecular genetics, proteomics) bear witness to our increasing ability to discover new drugs and the promise of identifying more and more drug receptors that will facilitate new modes of pharmacological therapy. That is the good news. The bad news concerns the rapidly escalating costs of drug development. It was noted in Chapter 1 that a reasonable estimate of the cost of developing a new drug in 2007 (the year of this book's publication) is on the order of US$1 billion dollars. This astronomical figure has less-than-attractive ramifications. Rawlins (2004) expressed the view that the increasing cost of drug development is likely to promote the situation whereby companies only invest in the development of drugs that are expected to recoup the research and development costs of the drug, which may necessitate peak annual sales on the order of US$500 million. In this context, he also observed:

> It is also worth noting that completely novel drug development—that is, against unproven disease targets—poses a greater risk of failure than developing drugs against proven targets. This provides additional incentive for companies to focus on improving on approaches that have been clinically and financially successful, and a disincentive to develop products for unmet medical needs. If

> the pharmaceutical industry's R&D efforts become concentrated solely on high-selling products, the outlook in many areas of pharmacotherapy—in particular those in which the risk of failure is high—is bleak (pp. 360-361).

Not surprisingly, following these comments, the author expressed the very reasonable view that "it is now imperative to make major efforts in reducing the costs of bringing new drugs to market" (Rawlins, 2004). While there are many other considerations in lowering these costs (e.g., terminating likely failures as early as possible, making manufacturing more cost-effective), Rawlins focused on potential cost-effective modifications of current regulatory requirements (see Rawlins, 2004, for additional discussion).

14.10 FDA's Critical Path Report and Critical Path Opportunities List

In March 2004, the FDA released its Critical Path Report and subsequently released its Critical Path Opportunities List in March 2006. The 2004 report discussed the "pipeline problem," the slowdown in innovative medical therapies reaching patients, and invited comments and suggestions from public and private stakeholders. Stakeholder response was considerable and positive, suggesting that the FDA "undertake research, develop guidances, initiate collaborations, and convene consensus-developing activities on a wide range of scientific issues." These suggestions were well received by the FDA. Their subsequent Critical Path Opportunities List, regarded as an initial summary of key scientific opportunities to improve product development, identifies targeted research that the FDA believes, if pursued, "will increase efficiency, predictability, and productivity in the development of new medical products." As the report noted:

> New scientific discoveries are not easily transformed into medical products, ready to treat new patients. Painstaking scientific work is needed to take a new laboratory discovery and turn it into a high-quality product that is beneficial and safe. Along this *Critical Path* are an array of difficult scientific and technological hurdles for medical product developers that are very different from the scientific challenges encountered in discovery.

The six topics that form the basis for the opportunities list are:

- Better evaluation tools—Developing new biomarkers and disease models.
- Streamlining clinical trials, including advancing innovative trial designs (as discussed in Chapter 11).
- Harnessing bioinformatics.

- ➢ Moving manufacturing into the twenty-first century, including the challenges in characterization, manufacturing, and quality assessment for combination products.
- ➢ Developing products to address urgent public health needs, including new antibiotics, vaccines, and medical countermeasures against emerging infections and bioterrorism attacks (see Grey and Spaeth, 2006, Roy, 2004).
- ➢ At-risk populations—Pediatrics.

Pediatric populations were discussed earlier when discussing several special populations (recall Section 10.12). As the FDA noted in this report:

> Children's bodies are not just small versions of adult bodies. Modifying the adult dose of a medicine might not result in the safe and effective treatment of a child. Ethical issues surrounding testing products in children often mean that children are faced with using devices, drugs, and biological products that have been rigorously tested only in adults. Critical Path research in these areas could help alleviate the twin problems of developing medical products for children and adolescents that address their unique physiologies and the uncertain ethics of testing products in these populations.

The FDA acknowledged that any new standards coming from the Critical Path Initiative should replace old standards, not constitute new requirements. As they noted, "The goal of the Critical Path Initiative is to modernize standards, not create roadblocks." Some regulatory actions that could contribute to more efficient product development included:

- ➢ Create the opportunity for more meetings with FDA staff earlier in the development process.
- ➢ Improve the consistency of FDA policies and procedures both within and across divisions and over time.
- ➢ Create more venues for collaboration with the FDA.
- ➢ Improve staffing levels and staffing continuity.
- ➢ Accelerate guidance document development (recall related discussion in Section 11.9.3).

The fourth item in this list, improve staffing levels and staffing continuity, is of interest for two reasons. Increasing staffing levels, at least in part, depends on increasing funds available to the FDA to pay employee salaries: Another part is attracting qualified employees. Improving staffing continuity is a related issue: It is advantageous (at the FDA as in many industries) to retain employees over time as they gain knowledge and experience and also build valuable professional relationships with sponsors and organizations with whom they work. In this context, further quotes from the IOM's (2006) recent report on the future of drug safety are illuminative:

> An agency whose crucial mission is to protect and advance the public's health should have adequate resources to do its job. The effect on CDER's work of CDER's overdependence on PDUFA [Prescription Drug User Fee Act] funding with restrictions on how FDA can use the money from user fees hurts FDA's credibility and may affect the agency's effectiveness.

PDUFA funds are those paid by a sponsor each time a regulatory application is submitted (see Mannebach et al., 2006). Currently, this constitutes a sizeable percentage of FDA's financial resources. The IOM report continues:

> To support improvements in drug safety and efficacy activities over a product's lifecycle, the committee recommends that the Administration should request and Congress should approve substantially increased resources in both funds and personnel for FDA. The committee favors appropriations from general revenues, rather than user fees, to support the full spectrum of new drug safety responsibilities proposed in this report.

14.11 COMING FULL CIRCLE: REVISITING THE BOOK'S "OPENING QUOTES"

As stated in Section 1.3, in the context of this book, the discipline of Statistics is regarded as a wide-ranging discipline that provides critical assistance in study design at all stages of new drug development and provides information that facilitates decision-making at all stages of this process. Throughout the book, statistical considerations were presented conceptually rather than computationally. In this penultimate section, it is appropriate to revisit these thoughts and to repeat my hope that, by now, the word "statistics" may appear less mysterious, irrelevant, or threatening to readers for whom the very mention of the word initially conjured up these or similar feelings.

In this context, I would also like to mention the six "Opening Quotes" provided at the front of this book. These quotes capture the essence of this book's discussions very well. At this point I invite you to read them again and to see how each one brings various aspects of our discussions to mind.

14.12 CONCLUDING COMMENTS

One major goal of this book has been to illustrate the central role of numerical representations of information in the process of new drug development. Accordingly, it has highlighted the roles of study design, experimental methodology, and statistical analysis in the areas of drug discovery, nonclinical research, preapproval clinical trials, and postmarketing surveillance. Emphasis has been placed on the roles of good design and good methodology in providing optimum quality data for analysis, interpretation, and use in decision making.

In addition to considering study design, experimental methodology, and statistical analysis, the book's chapters have discussed some of the operational activities and other influences on the work involved in new drug development. As we have seen, new drug development requires attention be paid to ethical, intellectual, scientific, biological, clinical, organizational, regulatory, financial, legal, congressional, social, and political considerations, and this list is likely far from exhaustive.

A second goal has been to illustrate that all of the activities described in this book are ultimately conducted to improve patients' health and well-being by changing their biology for the better. It is appropriate to remind ourselves frequently that our work has a very real impact on patients' lives. New drug development is a very complicated and difficult undertaking, but one that makes an enormous difference to the health of people across the globe. It is a noble pursuit.

If you work in this field, might be interested in doing so in the future, or have read this book because of your interest in clinical medicine, I hope it has helped you to have an appreciation of the central role of design, methodology, and analysis in new drug development and the importance of every professional's contribution to this process. I also hope the book has served to illustrate the nature of new drug development, the critical role of numerical representations of information in making informed decisions, and the central importance of biological and clinical considerations.

Appendix

Additional Resources for Training Executives and Professors

The following suggestions are respectfully offered as potential additional resources for training executives and professors who are interested in using this book. Training executives in pharmaceutical/biopharmaceutical companies and contract research organizations may wish to use this book as an introduction to new drug development in training programs for entry-level professionals and for professionals who wish to learn more about the central role of study design, experimental methodology, and statistical analysis in this process. Professors may wish to use it for courses on new drug development and study design and analysis in the context of pharmaceutical clinical trials. In both cases, the resources listed here may provide helpful complementary material to instructors.

The book by Steven Piantadosi, MD, PhD, is a definitive text on clinical trial methodology, and those by Gallin and Schuster and Powers are definitive books on clinical research. Those by Nally and Mann and Andrews similarly address two other topics covered in this volume, namely pharmaceutical manufacturing and pharmacovigilance. I recommend these books as main resources. The supplemental materials have been chosen since they provide accessible, compact, and affordable resources from which a wide range of topics can readily be taken. Additionally, training executives and professors may wish to choose one or more of these as recommended additional reading for their specific target audiences. Finally, one web site that is particularly informative about clinical trials is listed and an example of an FDA "Guidance for Industry" is provided.

Also, as noted in the Preface, a set of PowerPoint slides associated with this book is also available from the publisher's website for this book.

New Drug Development: Design, Methodology, and Analysis. By J. Rick Turner

MAIN RESOURCES

Gallin, J.I. (Ed), 2002, *Principles and practice of clinical research*, Academic Press.

Mann, R. and Andrews, E., (Eds), 2007, *Pharmacovigilance,* 2nd edition, John Wiley & Sons.

Nally, J.D., (Ed), 2006, *Good manufacturing practices for pharmaceuticals,* 6th edition, CRC Press.

Piantadosi, S., 2005, *Clinical trials: A methodologic perspective,* 2nd edition, Wiley-Interscience.

Schuster, D.P. and Powers, W.J. (Eds), 2005, *Translational and experimental clinical research*, Lippincott Williams & Wilkins.

SUPPLEMENTAL MATERIALS

Augen, J., 2005, *Bioinformatics in the post-genomic era: Genome, transcriptome, proteome, and information-based medicine,* Addison-Wesley (388 pages, paperback).

Bowers, D., House, A., and Owens, D., 2006, *Understanding clinical papers,* 2nd edition, John Wiley & Sons (232 pages, paperback).

Cobert, B., 2007, *Manual of drug safety and pharmacovigilance*, Jones and Bartlett (292 pages, paperback).

Derenzo, E. and Moss, J., 2006, *Writing clinical research protocols: Ethical considerations,* Elsevier/Academic Press (300 pages, paperback).

Fletcher, R.H. and Fletcher, S.W., 2005, *Clinical epidemiology,* 4th edition, Lippincott Williams & Wilkins (252 pages, paperback).

Machin, D. and Campbell, M.J., 2005, *Design of studies for medical research,* John Wiley & Sons (274 pages, paperback).

Matthews, J.N.S., 2006, *Introduction to randomized controlled clinical trials,* 2nd edition, Chapman & Hall/CRC (283 pages, paperback).

Mayer, D., 2004, *Essential evidence-based medicine*, Cambridge University Press (381 pages, paperback).

Mulder, G.J. and Dencker, L. (Eds), 2006, *Pharmaceutical toxicology*, Pharmaceutical Press (257 pages, paperback).

Primrose, S.B. and Twyman, R.M., 2004, *Genomics: Applications in human biology,* Blackwell Publishing (216 pages, paperback).

Rang, H.P. (Ed), 2006, *Drug discovery and development: Technology in transition,* Elsevier (346 pages, paperback).

Thomas, G., 2003, *Fundamentals of medicinal chemistry,* John Wiley & Sons (285 pages, paperback).

Tozer, T.N. and Rowland, M., 2006, *Introduction to pharmacokinetics and pharmacodynamics: The quantitative basis of drug therapy,* Lippincott Williams & Wilkins (326 pages, paperback).

Webb, P., Bain, C., and Pirozzo, S., 2005, *Essential epidemiology: An introduction for students and health professionals,* Cambridge University Press (355 pages, paperback).

WEBSITES

This web site, a service of the United States National Institutes of Health, provides "regularly updated information about federally and privately supported clinical research in human volunteers. ClinicalTrials.gov gives you information about a trial's purpose, who may participate, locations, and phone numbers for more details," http://www.clinicaltrials.gov.

FDA Guidance for Industry, March 2005, Good pharmacovigilance practices and pharmacoepidemiologic assessment, www.fda.gov/cder/guidance/6359OCC.htm.

A comprehensive list of FDA guidances can be found at http://www.fda.gov/cder/guidance/index.htm.

References

Ascione, F.J., 2001, *Principles of scientific literature evaluation: Critiquing clinical drug trials*, American Pharmaceutical Association.

Ashley, C., 2006, Clinical pharmacokinetics in renal impairment. In Dhillon, S. and Kostrzewski, A. (Eds), *Clinical pharmacokinetics*, Pharmaceutical Press, 53-77.

Augen, J., 2005, *Bioinformatics in the post-genomic era: Genome, transcriptome, proteome, and information-based medicine,* Addison-Wesley.

Bader, G.D. and Enright, A.J., 2005, Intermolecular interactions and biological pathways. In Baxevanis, A.D. and Ouellette, B.F.F. (Eds), *Bioinformatics: A practical guide to the analysis of genes and proteins, 3rd Edition,* Wiley-Interscience, 254-255.

Banks, M.N., Cacace, A.M., O'Connell, J., and Houston, J.G., 2005, High-throughput screening: Evolution of technology and methods. In Gad, S.C. (Ed), *Drug discovery handbook,* Wiley-Interscience, 559-602.

Becker, K.M. and Whyte, J.J. (Eds), 2006, *Clinical evaluation of medical devices: Principles and case studies, 2nd Edition,* Humana Press.

Berger, V.W., 2005, *Selection bias and covariate imbalances in randomized clinical trials,* John Wiley & Sons.

Blume, J. and Peipert, J.F., 2003, What your statistician never told you about *P*-values, *Journal of the American Association of Gynecologic Laparoscopists*, 10: 439-444.

Bond, C., (Ed), 2004, *Concordance*, Pharmaceutical Press.

Bosworth, H.B., Weinberger, M., and Oddone, E.Z., 2006a, Introduction. In Bosworth, H.B., Oddone, E.Z., and Weinberger, M. (Eds), *Patient treatment adherence: Concepts, interventions, and measurements*, Lawrence Erlbaum Associates, 3-11.

Bourne, H.R. and von Zastrow, M., 2004, Drug receptors and pharmacodynamics. In Katzung, B.G. (Ed), *Basic & clinical pharmacology, 9th Edition*, McGraw-Hill, 11-33.

New Drug Development: Design, Methodology, and Analysis. By J. Rick Turner

Bowers, A., 2005, Cracking the code of US federal regulations. *Regulatory Rapporteur*, 2(3): 6-11.

Bowers, D., House, A., and Owens, D., 2006, *Understanding clinical papers, 2nd Edition,* John Wiley & Sons.

Braeckman, R., 2005, Pharmacokinetics/ADME of large molecules. In Rogge, M.C. and Taft, D.R., (Eds), *Preclinical drug development.* Taylor & Francis, 159-198.

Brown, S.M., 2003, *Essentials of medical genomics,* Wiley-LISS.

Brun, P., 2006, Blinding of drug products. In Monkhouse, D.C., Carney, C.F., and Clark, J.L., (Eds), *Drug products for clinical trials, 2nd Edition,* Taylor & Francis, 149-172.

Bryson, B., 2003, *A short history of nearly everything,* Black Swan.

Buncher, C.R. and Tsay, J-Y., 2006a, Clinical trial designs. In Buncher, C.R. and Tsay, J-Y., (Eds), *Statistics in the pharmaceutical industry, 3rd Edition,* Chapman & Hall/CRC, 79-90.

Buncher, C.R. and Tsay, J-Y., 2006b, Phase IV postmarketing studies. In Buncher, C.R. and Tsay, J-Y., (Eds), *Statistics in the pharmaceutical industry, 3rd Edition,* Chapman & Hall/CRC, 303-314.

Cairns, C., 2006, Clinical pharmacokinetics in the elderly. In Dhillon, S. and Kostrzewski, A., (Eds), *Clinical pharmacokinetics,* Pharmaceutical Press, 99-114.

Campbell, M.J. and Machin, D., 1999, *Medical statistics: A commonsense approach, 3rd Edition,* John Wiley & Sons.

Campbell, M.K., Elbourne, D.R., Altman, D.G., for the CONSORT Group, 2004, CONSORT statement: Extension to cluster randomised trials, *British Medical Journal*, 328:702-708.

Chevret, S., (Ed), 2006, *Statistical methods for dose-finding experiments,* John Wiley & Sons.

Chorghade, M.S., 2006, Preface. In Chorghade, M.S., (Ed), *Drug discovery and development: Volume 1, Drug discovery,* Wiley-Interscience, xv-xix.

Chow, S-C. and Chang, M., 2007, *Adaptive design methods in clinical trials*, Chapman & Hall/CRC.

Chow, S-C., Chang, M., and Pong, A., 2005, Statistical consideration of adaptive methods in clinical development, *Journal of Biopharmaceutical Statistics,* 15: 575-591.

Chow, S-C. and Liu, J-P., 2004, *Design and analysis of clinical trials: Concepts and methodologies*, Wiley-Interscience.

Chow, S-C., Shao, J., and Wang, H., 2003, *Sample size calculations in clinical research,* CRC/Taylor Francis.

Chuang-Stein, C., 1992, Summarizing laboratory data with different reference ranges in multi-center clinical trials, *Drug Information Journal*, 26: 77-84.

Cook, S., 2004, *Clinical studies management: A practical guide to success*, CRC Press.

Derenzo, E. and Moss, J., 2006, *Writing clinical research protocols: Ethical considerations,* Elsevier.

Deverka, P. and Magnus, D., 2005, From genome to drug: Ethical issues. In Handen, J.S. (Ed), *Industrialization of drug discovery: From target selection through lead optimization,* Taylor & Francis, 245-289.

Dhillon, S. and Gill, K., 2006, Basic pharmacokinetics. In Dhillon, S. and Kostrzewski, A. (Eds), *Clinical pharmacokinetics,* Pharmaceutical Press, 1-44.

Dodson, K.L. and Abendschein, D.R., 2005, Presenting data in manuscripts. In Schuster, D.P. and Powers, W.J. (Eds), 2005, *Translational and experimental clinical research*, Lippincott Williams & Wilkins, 308-319.

Dolfini, D.M. and Tiano, F.J., 2006, Clinical supply packaging. In Monkhouse, D.C., Carney, C.F., and Clark, J.L., (Eds), *Drug products for clinical trials, 2nd Edition,* Taylor & Francis, 311-352.

Donahue, R.M.J. and Ruberg, S.J., 1997, Standardizing clinical study designs for accelerating drug development, *Drug Information Journal*, 31: 655-663.

Dubey, S.D., Chi, G.Y.H., and Kelly, R.E., 2006, The FDA and the IND/NDA statistical review process. In Buncher, C.R. and Tsay, J-Y., (Eds), *Statistics in the pharmaceutical industry, 3rd Edition,* Chapman & Hall/CRC, 55-78.

El-Haik, B. and Al-Aomar, R., 2006, *Simulation-based Lean Six-Sigma and design for Six-Sigma,* John Wiley & Sons.

Ellenberg, S.S., Fleming, T.R., and DeMets, D.L., 2003, *Data monitoring committees in clinical trials: A practical perspective,* John Wiley & Sons.

Evanoff, B., 2005, Reducing bias. In Schuster, D.P. and Powers, W.J. (Eds), *Translational and experimental clinical research,* Lippincott Williams & Wilkins, 67-72.

Ferkol, T., Israel, E., and Wechsler, M., 2005, Gene therapy and pharmacogenomic studies. In Schuster, D.P. and Powers, W.J. (Eds), *Translational and experimental clinical research,* Lippincott Williams & Wilkins.

Fischer, J. and Ganellin, C.R. (Eds), 2006, *Analogue-based drug discovery,* Wiley-VCH.

Fletcher, R.H. and Fletcher, S.W., 2005, *Clinical epidemiology, 4th Edition,* Lippincott Williams & Wilkins.

Florence, A.T. and Attwood, D., 2006, *Physiochemical principles of pharmacy, 4th Edition,* Pharmaceutical Press.

Fowler, J., Jarvis, P., and Chevannes, M., 2002, *Practical statistics for nursing and health care: A modern introduction*, John Wiley & Sons.

Friedman, L.M., Furberg, C.D., and DeMets, D.L., 2006, *Fundamentals of clinical trials, 3rd Edition*, Springer.

Gad, S.C., 2006, *Statistics and experimental design for toxicologists and pharmacologists, 4th Edition,* CRC Press.

Gallin, J.I. (Ed), 2002a, *Principles and practice of clinical research,* Academic Press.

Gallin, J.I., 2002b, A historical perspective on clinical research. In Gallin, J.I. (Ed), *Principles and practice of clinical research,* Academic Press, 1-11.

Gardner, M.J. and Altman, D.G., 1986, Estimation rather than hypothesis testing: Confidence intervals rather than *p*-values. In Gardner, M.J. and Altman, D.G. (Eds), *Statistics with confidence*, British Medical Association.

Good, P.I., 2006, *A manager's guide to the design and conduct of clinical trials, 2nd Edition,* Wiley-LISS.

Grabowski, H., 2006, Patents and new product development in the pharmaceutical and biotechnology industries. In Smith, C.G. and O'Donnell, J.T. (Eds), *The process of new drug discovery and development, 2nd Edition,* Informa Healthcare, 533-546.

Grey, M.R. and Spaeth, K.R., 2006, *The bioterrorism sourcebook*, McGraw Hill.

Hagglof, I. and Holmgren, A., 2006, Regulatory affairs. In Rang, H.P. (Ed), *Drug discovery and development: Technology in transition,* Elsevier, 281-297.

Hansten, P.D., 2004, Appendix II: Important drug interactions and their mechanisms. In Katzung, B.G. (Ed), *Basic & clinical pharmacology, 9th Edition*, McGraw-Hill, 1110-1124.

Hartl, D.L. and Jones, E.W., 2006, *Essential genetics: A genomics perspective, 4th Edition,* Jones and Bartlett.

Hauschke, D., Steinijans, V., and Pigeot, I., 2007, *Bioequivalence studies in drug development: Methods and applications*, John Wiley & Sons.

Haynes, R.B., Sackett, D.L., Guyatt, G.H., and Tugwell, P., 2006, *Clinical epidemiology: How to do clinical practice research, 3rd edition,* Lippincott Williams & Wilkins.

Hellman, B., 2006, General toxicology. In Mulder, G.J. and Dencker L. (Eds), *Pharmaceutical toxicology*, Pharmaceutical Press, 1-39.

Ho, R.J.Y. and Gibaldi, G., 2003, *Biotechnology and biopharmaceuticals: Transforming proteins and genes into drugs,* Wiley-LISS.

Holmes, M.R., Ramkissoon, K.R., and Giddings, M.C., 2005, Proteomics and protein identification. In Baxevanis, A.D. and Ouellette, B.F.F. (Eds), *Bioinformatics: A practical guide to the analysis of genes and proteins, 3rd Edition,* Wiley-Interscience, 445-472.

Homon, C.A. and Nelson, R.M., 2006, High-throughput screening: Enabling and influencing the process of drug discovery. In Smith, C.G. and O'Donnell, J.T. (Eds), *The process of new drug discovery and development, 2nd Edition,* Informa Healthcare, 79-102.

Hudes, G., Menon, S., and Golemis, E.A., 2004, Protein interaction-targeted drug discovery. In Rapley, R. and Harbron, S. (Eds), *Molecular analysis and genome discovery*, John Wiley & Sons, 323-345.

Hung, H.M.J., O'Neill, R.T., Wang, S-J., and Lawrence, J., 2006, A regulatory view on adaptive/flexible clinical trial design, *Biometrical Journal*, 48: 565-573.

Hwang, I.K. and Lan, K.K.G., 2006, Interim analysis and adaptive design in clinical trials. In Buncher, C.R. and Tsay, J-Y. (Eds), *Statistics in the pharmaceutical industry, 3rd Edition,* Chapman & Hall/CRC, 245-284.

ICH Guideline E1: The extent of population exposure to assess clinical safety for drugs intended for long-term treatment of non-life-threatening conditions. (See www.ich.org.)

ICH Guideline E2A: Clinical safety data management: Definitions and standards for expedited reporting. (See www.ich.org.)

ICH Guideline E6 (R1): Guideline for good clinical practice. (See www.ich.org.)

ICH Guideline E8: General consideration of clinical trials. (See www.ich.org.)

ICH Guideline E9: Statistical principles for clinical trials. (See www.ich.org.)

ICH Guideline E10: Choice of control group and related issues in clinical trials. (See www.ich.org.)

ICH Guideline M3(R1): Non-clinical safety studies for the conduct of human clinical trials for pharmaceuticals. (See www.ich.org.)

ICH Guideline M4: The common technical document. (See www.ich.org.)

ICH Guideline Q1A(R2): Stability testing of new drug substances and products. (See www.ich.org.)

ICH Guideline Q1E: Stability data evaluation. (See www.ich.org.)

ICH Guideline S3B: Pharmacokinetics: Guidance for repeated dose tissue distribution studies. (See www.ich.org.)

Jones, D., 2002, *Pharmaceutical statistics*, Pharmaceutical Press.

Jones, S.D. and Warren, P.G., 2006, Proteomics and drug discovery. In Chorghade, M.S. (Ed), *Drug discovery and development: Volume 1, Drug discovery,* Wiley-Interscience, 233-271.

Kalow, W., 2005, Historical aspects of pharmacogenetics. In Kalow, W., Meyer, U.A., and Tyndale, R.F. (Eds), *Pharmacogenomics, 2nd Edition,* Taylor & Francis, 1-11.

Kannel, W.B. and Sorlie P., 1975, Hypertension in Framingham. In Paul, O. (Ed), *Epidemiology and control of hypertension*, Grune & Stratton/Intercontinental Medical Book Corporation.

Katz, D.L., 2001, *Clinical epidemiology & evidence-based medicine: Fundamental principles of clinical reasoning & research,* Sage Publications.

Kay, R., 2005, Statistical thinking in clinical trials. Course given to GlaxoSmithKline Clinical Submissions Management employees, Chapel Hill, NC, May 2005.

Koren, G., 2004, Special aspects of perinatal and pediatric pharmacology. In Katzung, B.G. (Ed), *Basic & clinical pharmacology, 9th Edition*, McGraw-Hill, 995-1006.

Krauss, G., 2003, *Biochemistry of signal transduction and regulation, Third, Completely revised edition,* Wiley-VCH.

Krupa, J., 2006, Project management. In Monkhouse, D.C., Carney, C.F., and Clark, J.L. (Eds), *Drug products for clinical trials, 2nd Edition,* Taylor & Francis, 353-389.

Lednicer, D., 2007, *New drug discovery and development,* Wiley-Interscience.

Lesko, L.J., Salerno, R.A., Spear, B.B., *et al.,* 2006, Pharmacogenetics and pharmacogenomics in drug development and regulatory decision-making: Report of the first FDA-PWG-PhRMA-DruSafe Workshop. In Smith, C.G. and O'Donnell, J.T. (Eds), *The process of new drug discovery and development, 2nd Edition,* Informa Healthcare, 199-223.

Lesko, L.J. and Woodcock, J., 2005, Regulatory perspectives on pharmacogenomics. In Kalow, W., Meyer, U.A., and Tyndale, R.F. (Eds), *Pharmacogenomics, 2nd Edition,* Taylor & Francis, 265-286.

LeVine, H., 2006, Biopharmaceuticals. In Rang, H.P. (Ed), *Drug discovery and development: Technology in transition,* Elsevier, 177-194.

Liu, Q. and Pledger, G., 2006, Interim analysis and bias in clinical trials: The adaptive design perspective. In Buncher, C.R. and Tsay, J-Y. (Eds), *Statistics in the pharmaceutical industry, 3rd Edition,* Chapman & Hall/CRC, 231-244.

Loregian, A. and Palu, G., 2005, Strategies and methods in monitoring and targeting protein-protein interactions. In Gad, S.C. (Ed), *Drug discovery handbook,* Wiley-Interscience.

Machin, D. and Campbell, M.J., 2005, *Design of studies for medical research,* John Wiley & Sons.

Mannebach, A., Ward, M., and Adkins, B., 2006, Reviewing the Prescription Drug User Fee Act (PDUFA), *Regulatory Rapporteur*, September 2006, 12-16.

Matthews, J.N.S., 1999, Preface. *Introduction to randomized controlled clinical trials,* Edward Arnold.

Matthews, J.N.S., 2006, *Introduction to randomized controlled clinical trials, 2nd Edition,* Chapman & Hall/CRC.

Mayer, D., 2004, *Essential evidence-based medicine*, Cambridge University Press.

Meibohm, B., 2006, The role of pharmacokinetics and pharmacodynamics in the development of biotech drugs. In Meibohm, B. (Ed), *Pharmacokinetics and pharmacodynamics of biotech drugs: Principles and case studies in drug development,* Wiley-VCH, 3-13.

Meyer, U.A., 2002, Introduction to pharmacogenomics: Promises, opportunities, and limitations. In Licinio, J. and Wong M-L. (Eds), *Pharmacogenomics: The search for individualized therapies,* Wiley-VCH, 1-8.

Mitscher, L.A. and Dutta A., 2006, Contemporary drug discovery. In Chorghade, M.S., (Ed), *Drug discovery and development: Volume 1, Drug discovery,* Wiley-Interscience. 103-128.

Moher, D., Schulz, K.F., Altman, D., for the CONSORT Group, 2001, The CONSORT Statement: Revised recommendations for improving the quality of reports of parallel-group randomized trials, *Journal of the American Medical Association*, 285: 1987-1991.

Molenberghs, G. and Kenward, M., 2007, *Missing data in clinical studies*, John Wiley & Sons.

Molzon, J.A., 2006, Common technical document: The changing face of the new drug application. In Smith, C.G. and O'Donnell, J.T. (Eds), *The process of new drug discovery and development, 2nd Edition,* Informa Healthcare, 473-479.

Monkhouse, D.C., 2006a, The clinical trials material professional: A changing role. In Monkhouse, D.C., Carney, C.F., and Clark, J.L. (Eds), *Drug products for clinical trials, 2nd Edition,* Taylor & Francis, 1-19.

Monkhouse, D.C., 2006b, Manufacturing and clinical medicine trends for the clinical trials material professional. In Monkhouse, D.C., Carney, C.F., and Clark, J.L. (Eds), *Drug products for clinical trials, 2nd Edition,* Taylor & Francis, 21-68.

Monkhouse, D.C., 2006c, Discovery and formulation trends for the clinical trials material professional. In Monkhouse, D.C., Carney, C.F., and Clark, J.L. (Eds), *Drug products for clinical trials, 2nd Edition,* Taylor & Francis, 69-110.

Mulder, G.J., 2006, Drug metabolism: Inactivation and activation of xenobiotics. In Mulder, G.J. and Dencker, L. (Eds), *Pharmaceutical toxicology*, Pharmaceutical Press, 41-66.

Mulvihill, D.A., Gibson, D.W., and Cole, T.G., 2005, Database development. In Schuster, D.P. and Powers, W.J. (Eds), *Translational and experimental clinical research,* Lippincott Williams & Wilkins, 113-121.

National Institutes of Health, U.S. Department of Health and Human Services, 2004, *The seventh report of the Joint National Committee [JNC 7] on prevention, detection, evaluation, and treatment of high blood pressure.* NIH Publication No. 04-5230.

Ng, R., 2004, *Drugs: From discovery to approval,* Wiley-LISS.

Nichol, F.R., 2006, Contract research organizations: Role and function in new drug development. In Smith, C.G. and O'Donnell, J.T. (Eds), *The process of new drug discovery and development, 2nd Edition,* Informa Healthcare, 407-418.

Nogrady, T. and Weaver, D.F., 2005, *Medicinal chemistry: A molecular and biochemical approach, 3rd Edition,* Oxford University Press.

Ofran, Y. and Rost, B., 2005, Predictive methods using protein sequences. In Baxevanis, A.D. and Ouellette, B.F.F. (Eds), *Bioinformatics: A practical guide to the analysis of genes and proteins, 3rd Edition,* Wiley-Interscience, 197-221.

Oliver, J.J. and Webb, D.J., 2003, Surrogate endpoints. In Wilkins, M.R. (Ed), *Experimental therapeutics*, Martin Dunitz/Taylor & Francis Group, 145-165.

Olsson, S. and Meyboom, R., 2006, Pharmacovigilance. In Mulder, G.J. and Dencker, L. (Eds), *Pharmaceutical toxicology*, Pharmaceutical Press.

O'Neill, R.T., 1987, Statistical analyses of adverse event data from clinical trials: Special emphasis on serious events, *Drug Information Journal*, 21: 9-20.

O'Neill, R.T., 2006, A regulatory perspective on data monitoring and interim analysis. In Buncher, C.R. and Tsay, J-Y. (Eds), *Statistics in the pharmaceutical industry, 3rd Edition,* Chapman & Hall/CRC, 285-293.

Pallay, A., 2000, A decision analytic approach to determining sample sizes in a Phase III program, *Drug Information Journal*, 34:365-377.

Patterson, S. and Jones, B., 2006, *Bioequivalence and statistics in clinical pharmacology,* Chapman & Hall/CRC.

Piaggio, G., Elbourne, D.R., Altman, D.G., Pocock, S.J., and Evans, S.J.W., for the CONSORT Group, 2006, Reporting of noninferiority and equivalence randomized trials: An extension of the CONSORT Statement, *Journal of the American Medical Association*, 295:1152-1160.

Piantadosi, S., 2005, *Clinical trials: A methodologic perspective, 2nd Edition,* Wiley-Interscience.

Popper, K., 2002, *The logic of scientific discovery,* Routledge Classics.

Primrose, S.B. and Twyman, R.M., 2004, *Genomics: Applications in human biology,* Blackwell Publishing.

Primrose, S.B. and Twyman, R.M., 2006, *Principles of gene manipulation and genomics, 7th Edition,* Blackwell Publishing.

Prokscha, S., 2007, *Practical guide to clinical data management, 2nd Edition,* Taylor & Francis.

Rang, H.P., 2006a, The development of the pharmaceutical industry. In Rang, H.P. (Ed), *Drug discovery and development: Technology in transition,* Churchill Livingstone/Elsevier, 3-18.

Rang, H.P., 2006b, The drug discovery process: General principles and some case histories. In Rang, H.P. (Ed), *Drug discovery and development: Technology in transition,* Churchill Livingstone/Elsevier, 45-56.

Rang, H.P. and LeVine, H., 2006, Therapeutic modalities. In Rang, H.P. (Ed), *Drug discovery and development: Technology in transition,* Churchill Livingstone/Elsevier, 33-40.

RAPS (Regulatory Affairs Professionals Society), 2005, *2005 Fundamentals of US regulatory affairs*, Regulatory Affairs Professionals Society.

Rawlins, M.D, 2004, Opinion: Cutting the cost of drug development, *Nature Reviews Drug Discovery*, 3: 360-364.

Roberts, R.J., 1993, An amazing distortion in DNA induced by a methyltransferase. Nobel Lecture (Nobel Prize for Medicine), December 8. (See http://nobelprize.org/nobel_prizes/medicine/laureates/1993/roberts-lecture.html, accessed November 14, 2006.)

Robinson, M. and Cook, S., 2005, *Clinical trials risk management*, CRC Press.

Rolan, P.E. and Molnar, V., 2006, The assessment of pharmacokinetics in early-phase drug evaluation. In Lee, C-J., Lee, L.H., Wu, C.L., Lee, B.R., and Chen, M-L. (Eds), *Clinical trials of drugs and biopharmaceuticals,* CRC/Taylor & Francis, 123-132.

Roses, A.D., 2004, Pharmacogenetics and drug development: The path to safer and more effective drugs. *Nature Reviews Genetics*, 5, 645-656.

Ross, N.T., McNaughton, B.R., and Miller, B.L., 2005, Combinatorial chemistry in the drug discovery process. In Gad, S.C. (Ed), *Drug discovery handbook,* Wiley-Interscience, 961-1011.

Rothstein, M.A. (Ed), 2003, Preface. *Pharmacogenomics: Social, ethical, and clinical dimensions*, Wiley-LISS.

Roy, M.J. (Ed), 2004, *Physician's guide to terrorist attack*, Humana Press.

Sackett, D.I., Rosenberg, W.M., Gray, J.A.M., Haynes, R.B., and Richardson, W.S., 1996, Evidence-based medicine: What it is and what it isn't, *British Medical Journal*, 312: 71-72.

Salek, S. and Edgar, A., (Eds), 2002, *Pharmaceutical ethics,* John Wiley & Sons.

Schuster, D.P., 2005, Introduction: The value of translational and experimental clinical research. In Schuster, D.P. and Powers, W.J. (Eds), *Translational and experimental clinical research,* Lippincott Williams & Wilkins, xv-xxi.

Schuster, D.P. and Powers, W.J. (Eds), 2005, *Translational and experimental clinical research,* Lippincott Williams & Wilkins.

Senn, S., 1997, *Statistical issues in drug development,* John Wiley & Sons.

Senn, S., 2002, *Cross-over trials in clinical research, 2nd Edition,* John Wiley & Sons.

Soloviev, M., Barry, R., and Terrett, J., 2004, Chip-based proteomics technology. In Rapley, R. and Harbron, S. (Eds), *Molecular analysis and genome discovery,* John Wiley & Sons.

Spiegelhalter, D.J., Abrams, K.R., and Myles, J.P., 2004, *Bayesian approaches to clinical trials and health-care evaluation,* John Wiley & Sons.

Straus, S.E., Richardson, W.S., Glasziou, P., and Haynes, R.B., 2005, *Evidence-based medicine: How to practice and teach EBM*, Elsevier.

Subrahmanyam, V.V. and Tonelli, A.P., 2005, Pharmacokinetics/ADME of small molecules. In Rogge, M.C. and Taft, D.R. (Eds), *Preclinical drug development*, Taylor & Francis, 99-158.

Thomas, G., 2003, *Fundamentals of medicinal chemistry,* John Wiley & Sons.

Tozer, T.N. and Rowland, M., 2006, *Introduction to pharmacokinetics and pharmacodynamics: The quantitative basis of drug therapy,* Lippincott Williams & Wilkins.

Tsong, Y., Chen, C-W., Chen, W.J., *at al.,* 2006, Stability studies of pharmaceuticals. In Buncher, C.R. and Tsay, J-Y. (Eds), *Statistics in the pharmaceutical industry, 3rd Edition,* Chapman & Hall/CRC, 391-419.

Turner, J.R., 1994, *Cardiovascular reactivity and stress: Patterns of physiological response,* Plenum Press.

Voorhees, J. and Scheipeter, M.E., 2005, Case report form development. In Schuster, D.P. and Powers, W.J. (Eds), *Translational and experimental clinical research,* Lippincott Williams & Wilkins, 122-135.

Walsh, G., 2003, *Biopharmaceuticals: Biochemistry and biotechnology,* John Wiley & Sons.

Watson, J.D., 2004, *DNA: The secret of life,* Alfred A. Knopf.

Watson, J.D. and Crick, F.H.C., 1953, Molecular structure of nucleic acids: A structure for deoxyribose nucleic acid. *Nature*, April 25, 737.

Webb, P., Bain, C., and Pirozzo, S., 2005, *Essential epidemiology: An introduction for students and health professionals,* Cambridge University Press.

Weeks, C. and Tomlin, M., 2006, The effects of liver dysfunction on pharmacokinetics. In Dhillon, S. and Kostrzewski, A. (Eds), *Clinical pharmacokinetics*, Pharmaceutical Press, 79-98.

Wermuth, C.G., 2006, Pharmacophores: Historical perspective and viewpoint from a medicinal chemist. In Langer, T. and Hoffman, R.D. (Eds), *Pharmacophores and pharmacophore searches*, Wiley-VCH, 3-13.

Wishart, D., 2005, Protein structure and analysis. In Baxevanis, A.D. and Ouellette, B.F.F., (Eds), *Bioinformatics: A practical guide to the analysis of genes and proteins, 3rd Edition,* Wiley-Interscience, 223-251.

Woodward, M., 2005, *Epidemiology: Study design and data analysis, 2nd Edition,* Chapman & Hall/CRC.

Wurst, T.A. and Guernsey, B.G., 2006, Drug development on rails, *Applied Clinical Trials*, 15:38-44.

Index

New Drug Development: Design, Methodology, and Analysis. By J. Rick Turner

E

F

S

T

About the Author

J. Rick Turner Ph.D., is an experimental research scientist who spent many years in the field of cardiovascular behavioral medicine, investigating the effects of stress on the cardiovascular system and the possible role of stress-induced responses in the etiology of cardiovascular disease. He has published 50 peer-reviewed papers and seven authored and edited books. His text *Cardiovascular Reactivity and Stress: Patterns of Physiological Response* (New York: Plenum Press, 1994), the first such book in its field, introduced the methodology of cardiovascular reactivity research to upper level undergraduate and graduate students. He has received two international research awards and is a Fellow of the Society of Behavioral Medicine. He also has considerable experience in the clinical research arena as a medical writer, working most recently as a clinical submissions scientist at GlaxoSmithKline.

Dr. Turner is the Chairman of the Department of Clinical Research, Campbell University School of Pharmacy. He is also the President and Director of Scientific Affairs at Turner Medical Communications LLC. His company provides medical writing services to pharmaceutical/biopharmaceutical companies and contract research organizations. The Turner Medical Communications website information is provided at the end of this book's Preface.

His interests include sports, music, traveling the world with his wife, Karen, writing books, and all things Italian.

New Drug Development: Design, Methodology, and Analysis. By J. Rick Turner